The Weight, Hypnotherapy and YOU

Weight Reduction Program

An NLP and Hypnotherapy Practitioner's Manual

Judith E. Pearson, Ph.D.

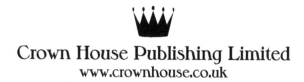

Crown House Publishing Limited
www.crownhouse.co.uk

First published by
Crown House Publishing Ltd
Crown Buildings, Bancyfelin, Carmarthen, Wales, SA33 5ND, UK
www.crownhouse.co.uk

and

Crown House Publishing Company LLC
PO Box 2223, Williston, VT 05495, USA
www.crownhousepublishing.com

Frst published 2006., reprinted 2007. Transferred to digital printing 2017.

British Library Cataloguing-in-Publication Data
A catalogue entry for this book is available from the British Library.

10-digit ISBN 1845900316
13-digit ISBN 978-1845900311

LCCN 2006929709

This book is dedicated to the memory of my mother,
Lois Jane Dyer Curtis.
She was my angel on earth. Now she is my angel in heaven.

The weight reduction program described in this book does not promise successful weight reduction for every client. It is not a cure for overeating or obesity nor a replacement or substitute for proper medical care and nutritional planning. No therapeutic program works with every client, and much of the success of the program described in this book rests in the skills of the practitioner and the motivation and personality of the client.

You are encouraged to view the WHY program as a working model that you can modify and improve upon according to your clinical judgment and the needs of your clients. The WHY program is not a franchise nor a "cookbook" program, and no promises or are made or implied as to any practitioner having increased income as a result of applying the program in his or her practice.

Contents

Acknowledgments

I owe the existence of this book to people who encouraged me, inspired me, gave me advice, and put up with me while I wrote it.

To my mentor, Ron Klein, founder and director of the American Hypnosis Training Academy in Silver Spring, Maryland, I express my heartfelt gratitude for his patient and methodical teachings in hypnotherapy and Neuro-Linguistic Programming (NLP). I took my first hypnotherapy training from Ron in 1988, and continued to attend his classes over the next four years, acquiring master's certification in NLP. I was deeply honored when he asked me to become an associate trainer, and under his supervision I obtained certification as an NLP trainer. Throughout our nearly two decades of friendship, he has consistently been a benevolent mentor, trusted colleague, and expert consultant to my practice. He is a teacher par excellence and a friend beyond measure.

I thank Kathy Corsetty, who invited me to coauthor *Healthy Habits* in 1998 and gave me permission to reprint and adapt from that work in writing this book. Having slimmed down by more than forty pounds, Kathy is a beautiful spirit and an inspiration to anyone who wishes to improve his or her health. She willingly shares her discoveries with others in a straightforward, unassuming way that instills hope and optimism. It is because of Kathy that I became interested in therapeutic approaches to weight control.

My gratitude goes to Dr. Jon Connelly, L.C.S.W.—a superb hypnotherapist and trainer, and the director of the Institute for Survivors of Sexual Violence, in Jupiter, Florida—who shared with me his thoughts and expertise on metaphors for addictions and compulsions. Our conversations explored the often-hidden meanings of words, language patterns, and symbolism. He gave me permission to capture many of those ideas in print in the final chapter of this book. I have learned much from Jon, and I admire his skill more than he will ever know.

I thank Dr. John Burton, Ed.D., a licensed professional counselor in private practice in Greenville, South Carolina, for inspiring me with his skills in Ericksonian hypnotherapy. John is a master practitioner of NLP and hypnotherapist extraordinaire who teaches others through his books on hypnotic language patterns. I revere his skills as a writer and therapist. John works with words in a manner that wields a gentle, trance-inducing power and imparts life-changing possibilities. I am touched and grateful that he agreed to write the foreword to this book.

Some special friends deserve mention. This book owes much to Carol Epner, R.N., a valued friend and colleague, as well as a registered nurse specializing in health and nutrition programs. She read the manuscript and gave me her expert advice on nutrition, medical issues, supplements, and obesity. Carol, bless you and thank you a thousand times for your generosity.

Retired clinical psychologist Joan Bartlett, Ph.D., a cherished friend, gave me tips and ideas from her many years of working in the field of hypnotherapy. We spent a few brief but memorable hours together one afternoon over soup and sandwiches in the Ritz Carlton lobby lounge in Arlington, Virginia, discussing the psychological aspects of obesity.

I could not have completed the section on audio recording if it were not for expert advice from Tom Goldsmith, husband of my friend Carol Goldsmith (a superb life coach and NLP practitioner), who was extraordinarily generous with his time and very patient with my ignorance about technical gadgets and computers. I also extend my thanks to Dr. Carl Arlotta, Ed.D., L.P.C.C., a counselor and hypnotherapist in Steubenville, Ohio, and former director of advising at Jefferson Community College, who pilot tested the scripts on two of his own clients in order to give me his feedback. Many warm thanks and regards to Dr. Rubin Battino, Ph.D., noted hypnotherapist, author, and professor emeritus at Wright State University, who devoted hours to critiquing the manuscript and gently prodding me to rework some of its rougher sections. I thank Gale Cohan, L.C.S.W., Gail Kalin, Ph.D., and Stephanie Tracy, L.C.S.W., psychotherapists and members of my monthly NLP discussion group, who encouraged me to write this book even before I thought of it. They kept up my spirits and motivation to complete the work.

To the staff of Crown House Publishing, I say thank you for believing that this book should and could become a reality. I very much appreciate your hospitality when I visited your offices in October 2005. It was my first trip through the green rolling countryside of Wales, a land of breathtaking beauty. I remember the thrill I felt when David Bowman told me that Crown House had accepted my book proposal. Since I began working with the staff, they have been patient, professional and have shown me every courtesy, understanding my novice standing as an author. I also appreciate the guidance and expertise of Kirsteen Anderson, freelance copyeditor, who polished the manuscript with me. I am sure she worked many hours on the task, despite her demanding family responsibilities.

My immeasurable appreciation goes to my husband, John Rodgaard, for his indefatigable support and encouragement. He tolerated my erratic sleeping and waking schedule while I worked on the manuscript and patiently endured my crabby moods when other duties delayed my progress. He was sympathetic when my computer misbehaved so frequently I finally had to replace it, only weeks before the manuscript was due. John was often a sounding board, lending a sanity check to my thinking. He cooked meals and attended to household chores to give me more time for writing. John was my chauffeur and travel companion on the trip to Wales to visit the staff at Crown House. He never doubted that this book would get into print. I have never doubted his love for me.

Finally, I thank my many clients who have shared with me their struggles and triumphs in weight management. Through our therapy sessions, they gave me their honesty, trust, and feedback, shaping my therapeutic approach and the vision for this book. I invite readers to improve upon the meager groundwork laid down in these pages, so that more people in the world are free from the burden of obesity.

Foreword

Wow, what a well-thought-out, in depth, and yet incredibly practical hypnotherapy program for weight loss! Judith Pearson's new book, which you are now holding, contains so much good information from so many practical realms. You can actually read this book and gain the necessary ingredients to utilize this effective weight loss program right now. More than just materials, resources, rationale, methods, and marketing, the whole program also rightly and naturally includes Judy's thoughtful compassion as a constant thread running through it.

I know quality work when I read it and Judy's is certainly top quality. I've worked for more than twenty years as a counselor and run my own counseling practice. I hold a doctorate in human development counseling and a master's in clinical psychology. Like Judy, I'm certified as a clinical hypnotherapist and a master practitioner of Neuro-Linguistic Programming (NLP). As a soon to be three-time published author, I am well aware of the rigors involved in conceiving the ideas, planning, and writing a manuscript, rewriting the manuscript and, oh, did I forget to mention, re-writing the manuscript. What I'm getting at is that completing a manuscript requires great commitment to the process of conveying ideas in a clear and useful manner. Judy has accomplished this daunting task to such a high degree that her thoroughness itself is worthy of high praise. And now I'll address the contents of her weight loss manual.

Any of us who have worked with clients on their eating habits and weight issues know how difficult this process can be. Clients with weight issues, overeating, and sedentary lifestyles often seek out hypnotherapists to assist in making changes happen. And when a television program airs that highlights the effective use of hypnosis in weight loss, well, you can be sure your phone will ring with calls from eager clients. But you may be at somewhat of a loss as to how to provide effective treatment.

Judy identifies all the issues I can imagine that are involved with starting and running a hypnotherapy program for weight loss. She details what you need to know and do before, during, and after the program to make it successful for your clients and yourself. This manual provides you with methods of marketing the program and developing your business. Judy also provides numerous dimensions of treatment within and around the actual hypnotherapy. She acknowledges and encourages the important elements of medical evaluations and nutritional awareness for the client. As you and I know, enlisting and informing clients increases motivation and positive outcomes.

Judy gives a plethora of intervention techniques to be used in session by the therapist as well as outside the sessions by the client. Certainly, the client is the most influential variable in any treatment outcome, regardless of the technique used. By providing intervention methods for the therapist *and* for the client to utilize on self, Judy ensures the maximum opportunity for success all the way around.

Part III contains a wealth of specific and general material. Judy presents very useful hypnotic language patterns geared for weight loss. She also cites great resources that allow you to find and learn more about constructing your own hypnotic language scripts tailored for the individual client. She details advanced language patterns and Sleight of Mouth, and displays mastery of these as well as NLP techniques.

You can utilize this collection of intervention tools as designed or use the general ingredients to create and apply interventions to suit your clients. You can even find that these general principles serve as a nice reminder about advanced language patterns in interventions with just about any client issue. Judy is so amazingly thorough that before I can even wonder beyond what I'm reading or ask a question, she answers it for me. She covers material as I start wondering, troubleshooting before trouble begins. I think that's known as prevention, which is very satisfying.

Chapter 17 presents wonderful information that provides the materials and "how to" for constructing effective metaphors. These materials can then be used for making and applying metaphors with clients' weight issues. But, again, these materials can also be used for constructing metaphors for use with other issues if you utilize the general principles. Again, great sources and resources come along with the specific material, allowing you to develop your skills further for weight loss clients and others.

Chapter 18 addresses very important matters that can often be overlooked. What will life be like after the change takes place? What skills will be needed to sustain these new ways? What issues might crop up that could undermine the progress and maintenance of them? What strategies might allow successful negotiating of these issues? These questions and their answers make crucial ingredients for any successful personal change. By anticipating old issues or old pivot points that will present in the future, the therapist and client can set out guiding lights, predetermined response sets that will steer the client along the successful path of health.

And for those who want to explore and understand the research that utilizes the various ingredients of effective weight loss, there exists a very fine set of appendixes. These present research that deals with the effects of exercise on body weight, hypnosis used for weight control, and brain health care factors that influence weight. Judy also includes ways to learn and utilize more advanced hypnotic skills and provides primers on clinical hypnosis and NLP.

Now you may choose to read this book, this comprehensive manual of a weight loss program in order to develop and run your own weight loss program for your clients. You may choose to read this manual for the specific information and intervention techniques. Or you may choose to read this book for the general dynamics and principles presented that make up potent personal change agents. Well, you can take it from here and enjoy the read for so many reasons.

John Burton, Ed.D.
Greenville, South Carolina

Preface

Imagine that you could help people who are overweight or obese achieve the weight they choose. Imagine you could offer them a proven program for weight reduction, incorporating your skills in hypnotherapy and Neuro-Linguistic Programming (NLP). Imagine making a significant difference in the lives of these people who, because of their weight problems, run the risk of life-threatening diseases and grapple with self-consciousness, embarrassment, restricted movement, clumsiness, and social disapproval.

Imagine the rewarding feeling of seeing your overweight clients getting slimmer and healthier! Imagine getting referrals from satisfied clients, as well as physicians and health-care clinics, while continuing to hone your expertise as a practitioner who gets results where others have failed. Nothing can quite match the gratifying feeling of hearing a now-slender client say, "You helped me find my motivation. I couldn't have done it without you. Thank you."

This is what has happened for me since I created the Weight, Hypnotherapy and YOU (WHY) Weight Reduction Program a few years ago. Let me give you one success story as an example. One of my most gratifying experiences occurred with Ben (not his real name). Ben lumbered into my office for his first appointment weighing probably between 250 and 300 pounds. He had an amiable personality, yet was somewhat lacking in self-confidence and was not particularly well dressed or groomed. He told me he was working in an auto body shop, but his real ambition was to become an agent with the Federal Bureau of Investigation (FBI). To qualify for the job, he would have to undergo rigorous physical and academic training in Quantico, Virginia. Ben had already met with the FBI recruiter and had passed the initial screening interview. His problem was his weight. He could not qualify unless he could reach and maintain a healthy weight.

I conducted a few NLP and hypnotherapy sessions with Ben, loosely based on some ideas I was pulling together for what would eventually become the WHY Weight Reduction Program. He began to change his eating habits and exercise more, and said he was starting to lose weight. I had audiotaped our sessions, and Ben said that listening to the tapes was really helping him change his habits. At the end of those few sessions, I said goodbye to Ben and applauded his progress. I doubted, however, that he was really FBI material.

About three years later Ben phoned and asked me if I remembered him, stating that he had come to me for weight reduction. I did remember him, but the image in my mind was of the overweight, awkward guy I had last seen. He explained he was about to take his final exam at the FBI training academy and asked if I could work with him, using hypnotherapy, to help his concentration. I was surprised and elated to hear that Ben was indeed graduating from the FBI program. That, however, was nothing compared to my utter astonishment when he arrived two days later for his appointment. In walked a totally different man—extremely good-looking (we're talking gorgeous here!), with the build of an athlete, brimming with confidence, well dressed, and affable. WOW! It was all I could think of to say. WOW!

When people who are overweight reach the weight they envision, it truly transforms every aspect of their lives. Watching it happen, and knowing you have had a hand in the process, is one of the most rewarding experiences you'll ever have as a practitioner.

Perhaps you've felt the same way as many other practitioners who are reluctant to work with clients who have weight issues. There are valid reasons why working with this population is daunting. First, they generally have a high failure rate when it comes to weight reduction. Second, obesity is usually a chronic, life-long problem. Third, relapses are frequent because the temptation to overeat or eat the wrong kind of food is ever-present. Fourth, with obesity, people tend to feel socially inept and self-conscious. They may easily and frequently become discouraged and depressed. They are often unattractive, lonely, unhappy people. Who wouldn't be, having to lug around an extra fifty or one hundred pounds of fat?

If you've ever doubted your ability to help clients with effective weight management, you are not alone. I once had the same reservations myself. Now that I have a method for working with people who are obese or overweight, I don't feel that way anymore. The WHY program gives me quite an advantage, because it allows me to serve a wider range of clients and expand my clientele. I want you to have that advantage, too.

You have in your hands a practitioner's manual for a structured yet flexible hypnotherapy program you can offer to your clients who are struggling with obesity and the challenges of a chronic weight problem. It is a tested program that can produce results if you follow the instructions in this manual.

Judith E. Pearson, Ph.D.
Springfield, Virginia

Part I

What You Need to Know before You Begin

Chapter 1

How the WHY Program Came into Existence

I developed the Weight, Hypnotherapy and YOU Program for my practice; I really didn't intend to write a book about it. I just wanted a hypnotherapy program to treat obesity. Obesity continues to present a major health problem for millions. Many of those millions are turning to brief, solution-oriented therapies, such as NLP and hypnotherapy, for a solution. Some years ago, when I decided I wanted to extend my counseling services to this population, I set out to investigate how other practitioners were addressing the problem.

I searched the Internet and found several companies offering sets of hypnosis audiotapes, but little else. The colleagues I talked with seemed to use an ad hoc approach, and many seemed just as daunted as I was about working with clients with weight issues. I could not find the sort of program I was looking for, so I ended up creating my own. I read books on the subject, I looked at relevant research studies, and I asked for ideas and feedback from clients and colleagues. Through trial and error, I came up with the WHY Program.

In this chapter, I will tell you how the program, and subsequently this book, came into existence, and what you'll find in these pages. First, however, let me tell you about the extent of the obesity problem, so you'll understand more about why it is so important for practitioners to have effective skills and methods for working with people who are overweight.

The Extent of the Problem

Obesity is a serious medical and social issue that affects millions of people. According to the Weight-control Information Network web site (2005), nearly two-thirds of adults in the U.S. are overweight, and 30.5 percent are obese (usually defined as forty or more pounds, or eighteen-plus kilos, over the recommended weight). The statistics are even higher for those of Hispanic or African heritage. Excess weight and obesity affect 129.6 million people in the United States alone. The prevalence of obesity more than doubled between 1960 and 2000, and has continued to increase.

The American Society of Bariatric Physicians (2005) regards obesity as a "chronic medical disease with serious health implications." The health risks related to obesity include heart disease, diabetes, high blood pressure, hypertension, stroke, sleep apnea, gout, osteoarthritis, joint problems, and gall bladder disease. Even some forms of cancer are associated with excess weight. Weight problems shorten life span and reduce mobility. Moreover, an overweight population is costing their employers and the insurance industry billions of dollars in medical costs and lost productivity due to weight-related illnesses. Here are some U.S. statistics:

- The total health-care and lost productivity costs attributable to obesity amounted to $99.2 billion in 1995. These costs encompassed hospitalization for weight-related illnesses and injuries, weight-related disability payments, and lost work days for sickness, hospitalization, doctor visits, recovery time, and disability.

- Approximately $51.65 billion of that amount were direct medical costs.

- The health-related economic cost of obesity to U.S. businesses is substantial, representing approximately 5 percent of total medical care costs.

- Obesity-related medical conditions contribute to 300,000 deaths each year.

There is every reason to believe these costs and statistics will continue to rise along with obesity rates. According to the U.S. Centers for Disease Control and Prevention (2005), obesity may soon overtake tobacco as the leading cause of preventable death in the United States. People are seeking remedies for their weight problems through medical interventions, nutritional counseling, fitness programs, alternative medicines, food supplements, diets, and prescription drugs. No wonder weight reduction products and services are rapidly becoming a big business!

Moreover, it isn't always health concerns that lead people to seek help in managing their weight. We are a society obsessed with physical beauty and attractiveness. We spend billions of dollars on good looks. We buy diet books, memberships to health spas and gyms, designer clothes, cosmetics, and cosmetic surgery. People are obviously willing to spend money on products and services that will enhance their appearance.

With favorable publicity about the efficacy of brief, solution-oriented therapies and a public more willing than ever to spend money on health and beauty, many individuals are turning to hypnotherapy and NLP for help with weight control. This practitioner's manual is for medical professionals and mental-health professionals who want to address the needs of an overweight client population.

How the WHY Program Began

Some years ago, when I completed my certification training in NLP and hypnotherapy, and began incorporating those skills into my psychotherapy practice, I did not anticipate that clients would be seeking my services for weight control. A few people saw my "hypnotherapist" ads in the telephone directory and called, asking if hypnosis would help them lose weight. I told them they would be better served by consulting their family physician and following a physician-recommended diet regimen. I really had no interest in working with obesity and regarded it as a chronic health problem that could not be solved with a few sessions of psychotherapy.

Then several factors came together to change my mind. First, beginning in the late 1990s, the media began running news stories about the extent of the obesity problem in prosperous nations. Let's face it: Those statistics represent a sizable portion of the population—and a sizable market for weight reduction services. It seemed to me that if scientific research showed hypnotherapy to have some efficacy for weight management, then perhaps I could find a way to work with that population.

At the same time as news headlines began to emerge about the obesity epidemic, a friend and colleague, Kathy Corsetty, asked me to coauthor a book about fitness and weight control. Kathy is an NLP practitioner, motivational speaker, former Dale Carnegie instructor, and founder of the Healthy Habits program, which teaches people healthy weight-management methods. While I was writing this book, Kathy gave me permission to share her story:

Kathy had been a yo-yo dieter until 1986, when she attended a Tony Robbins seminar that helped her discover many of the root causes of her weight problems.[1] The seminar employed many NLP techniques. Kathy decided to learn everything she could about health, nutrition, and the underlying causes of being overweight.

Once her motivation was charged up, she read more than 200 books on health and nutrition. She slimmed down gradually and safely. In 1993 she even participated in a triathlon, swimming one mile in open waters, riding a bike forty kilometers, and running a ten-kilometer race. Since then, she has kept the weight off successfully, even following a pregnancy. Kathy and I met in the mid-1990s at an NLP master practitioner certification training at the American Hypnosis Training Academy in Silver Spring, Maryland, where I occasionally work as an associate trainer. She asked me if I could help her write a book describing the NLP patterns that contribute to a healthy lifestyle.

That book, *Healthy Habits,* was published in 2000. Coauthoring that book taught me a great deal about nutrition and exercise and how to describe the factors that help people get into healthy physical condition. Kathy and I received positive feedback from our readers and, of course, a few readers became my clients.

While I could confidently say to my first few overweight clients, "Read the book," I didn't have much initial success in helping them reduce their weight. Here's what happened with Linda (not her real name). Each week Linda would come in for her one-hour session. She would present some behavioral problem related to food or overeating, and I would offer an NLP intervention that seemed appropriate. On other occasions I used more "traditional" hypnotic methods, taking her through a guided visualization or a metaphor, with direct and indirect suggestions about changes she could make with regard to eating and exercise. Although Linda was cooperative and our sessions together were warm and enjoyable, the fact was this: Linda was not reducing her weight. She seemed more interested in *talking* about her weight (she weighed about 250 pounds, or almost 114 kilograms) than doing anything meaningful about it.

I finally referred her to a nutritionist, who designed a nutritional plan for Linda's needs, gave her specific take-home assignments, and held her accountable for making progress. Guess what? Linda began shedding all that extra weight. When the same thing happened with a second client, I decided something was wrong with my approach. Perhaps I needed a more structured program. Perhaps I too could give clients take-home assignments and hold them accountable. "But, how?" I wondered.

I also wondered (as I have heard some experts theorize) whether compulsive eating has its basis in significant childhood events. For my next two clients, I focused the therapy sessions on underlying emotional conflicts and childhood events. Guess what? Both clients dropped out after the third session. The feedback I got was that the therapy was not addressing their day-to-day concerns about how to eat and how to have a healthy relationship with food. What did I learn? Although childhood events probably have some bearing on compulsive eating and obesity, I believe that clients as a rule are not interested in exploring the emotional origins of their eating patterns. They want practical solutions that directly address their daily behavior issues around weight, food, and exercise.

Reflecting on my lack of success, I doubted that NLP and hypnotherapy really had any efficacy for helping people get to a healthy weight and stay there. I began to investigate that question. I searched the Internet and university libraries for actual research. I was not convinced by testimonials on web sites and advertisements that seemed to be more hype than substance. I wanted evidence—not grandiose claims and wishful thinking. That's where another factor came in that convinced me to develop the WHY Program. I found medical studies suggesting that hypnotherapy could be effective in helping people reduce their weight when used in conjunction with other weight reduction methods such as behavioral therapy, exercise, and a low-fat diet. Every experimental study I read about employed a structured program of six to eight sessions of hypnotherapy. Appendix A contains abstracts of these studies. I also present the findings of those studies in report form in appendix B.

Based on the findings from those studies, I decided to develop a weight reduction program consisting of eight sessions of NLP counseling and hypnotherapy. After considering several names, I settled on the WHY acronym because this program is about weight, hypnotherapy, and YOU (i.e., the client). I wanted a name that was short and easy to remember, might arouse interest and curiosity, and didn't sound like a diet or weight-loss pill.

In designing the WHY Program, I incorporated many ideas from *Modern Clinical Hypnosis for Habit Control*, by Citrenbaum, King, and Cohen (1985), long considered a seminal text on hypnotherapy for treating smoking, overeating, and alcohol abuse. For habit control, the book offers hypnotherapists the following advice:

- Carefully screen clients, not only for motivation, but also for medical and psychological symptoms and contraindications.
- Acquire information and knowledge about the psychological aspects of habits and addictions, as well as the health risks of smoking, alcoholism, and obesity.
- Give clients a thorough explanation of the hypnotherapy process.
- Assist clients in reframing the unconscious positive intentions that destructive habits are seeking to fulfill.
- Observe ecological considerations unique to each client.
- Make creative use of metaphors, embedded suggestions, direct and indirect suggestions, and hypnotic language patterns in the hypnotherapy process.

Additionally, I reviewed my notes from clinical interviews with my weight-loss clients and talked to colleagues about their experiences with such clients. Patterns began to emerge. People who are overweight often

- eat according to external cues, not internal hunger signals
- eat for emotional comfort, regarding food as an antidote for any kind of emotional distress
- plan social activities around food
- reward themselves with food
- report that they were admonished as children not to waste food, to clean their plates, to eat to show appreciation to the person who cooked the meal, or to put on weight "in case you get sick"

- place little value on physical activity and are not often motivated to exercise
- maintain a self-image and identity as an overweight person and eat accordingly
- prefer sweet and fattening foods over those that offer balanced nutrition
- overeat because they do not understand correct portion size, do not control their portions, or both. They overeat beyond the point where other people would feel quite full and satiated. They do not experience or do not attend to the sensations of a full stomach
- eat unconsciously while doing other things—watching television, reading a book, talking on the phone, and the like
- feel discouraged when they think about how much weight they want to lose because they don't mentally chunk down the process to the task of losing one or two pounds (or one kilo) a week
- often have a dual diagnosis of compulsive eating and clinical depression
- think of dieting as a form of deprivation and starvation
- have followed several diets successfully, but when they reached their target weight, they discarded the diet and regained the weight
- do not know exactly how much they weigh because they are embarrassed to get on a scale and avoid doing so for months or sometimes years at a time
- do not realize how much food they eat in a day's time
- say they know everything there is about losing weight but often don't know basic information such as how many calories one has to burn to lose a single pound or a single kilo.

These patterns are not intended as stereotypes. Every client seems to have a unique combination of these behaviors and attitudes. Granted, slender people also have some these habits, but not to the extent of gaining and maintaining excessive amounts of weight. One overweight client told me, "My appetite doesn't seem to have an 'off' switch. I can't determine when I feel full and I don't know when to stop eating." Another told me, "I think of food day and night. Eating is all I want to do. I obsess about food." Another problem I hear very frequently is, "I eat for every emotion I feel, whether I feel happy or sad. If I feel sad, I eat for comfort. If I feel happy, I eat to celebrate." Slender people just do not think this way.

I was determined to develop an NLP and hypnotherapy program that would address the all-too-common behavioral-emotional problems of the population with obesity. I wanted a program based on a flexible structure of reliable methods through which clients would see actual weight reduction in a reasonable amount of time at a reasonable price. I spent several days mapping out a program that would combine all I had learned. I designed the program to meet my criteria for any good psychotherapy service: It must be ethical, safe, realistic, practical, and marketable, and it must deliver results.

When I started telling other practitioners I had a hypnotherapy program for weight reduction, they wanted to know more about it. When I described the program, they would scribble voluminous notes for a while, then throw up their hands and say, "This is too much to remember! You should put all of this in writing! Why don't you write a book?" So I decided to share the program with you by writing this book.

What You'll Find in This Book

This book is divided into three parts. The first, "What You Need to Know before You Begin," gives you preparatory information about the WHY Program. In chapter 2, I tell you about the success factors that went into the development of the WHY Program and how, with the "accountability factor," you can be sure clients *will* lose weight, yet at a safe rate in small increments. Chapter 3 gives you an overview of the WHY Program. It explains the general content (much of which you can change or adapt) of each of the eight sessions, the structure of the hypnotherapy scripts, the rationale for recording the sessions (either on audiotapes or CDs), contraindications (used for screening clients), helpful tips about language, and how to maintain your own flexibility in using the WHY Program. Chapter 4 discusses the professional skills you need to conduct the WHY program: your clinical skills, what you need to know about weight control and nutrition, your familiarity with community resources, how to make audio recordings, and how to set your fee. Chapter 5 provides a dozen ways to market the WHY Program for your own practice.

Part II, "Conducting the Eight Sessions of the WHY Program," lays out a completely scripted model of the WHY Program in chapters 6 to 13. In this section, I show you in detail how I conduct each of the eight sessions, with step-by-step instructions and sample scripts. Part II also has a "bonus," general-purpose script in chapter 14. As you acquire experience with implementing the eight sessions, I fully anticipate that you will adapt the methods and wording for your own preferences, uses, and purposes. The program offers plenty of flexibility for you to do so.

Part III, "Enhancing Success," chapters 15 through 20, suggests ways to increase your and your clients' success with the WHY Program. Chapter 15 gives guidance on working with "stuck" clients—those who are not making progress and may feel as though they want to give up and drop out of the program. Chapter 16 contains a host of additional NLP patterns for working with compulsive eating. Chapter 17 describes how to work with advanced language patterns. Chapter 18 has suggestions for follow-up sessions for clients who may benefit from additional mental-health-related services. Chapter 19 lists tough questions and honest, forthright answers about the WHY Program, ending with client testimonials. Chapter 20 is an interview with Dr. Jon Connelly, director of the Institute for Survivors of Sexual Violence, who offers some insightful observations on addictions and compulsive eating. You can find much valuable information in the appendixes as well.

This book is intended for licensed or certified psychotherapists, counselors, coaches, nutritionists, pastoral counselors, mental-health practitioners, social workers, nurses, physicians, psychiatrists, and medical practitioners who have certification training in NLP and hypnotherapy. I have included everything you need to know in order to conduct this eight-session hypnotherapy-based weight reduction program effectively and ethically. It is a structured program, yet you can tailor it to the needs of each client. Scientific research shows that hypnotherapy can help people manage their eating patterns and reduce their weight. The challenge for practitioners is to implement these findings. I am convinced the WHY Program is a worthwhile, marketable service that will produce rewards for your clients, satisfaction for you, and income for your practice.

Chapter 2

Factors Necessary for Success with the WHY Program

This chapter explains the factors that lead to success with the WHY Program. Every single factor is essential to helping you conduct this program successfully. In developing the program, I chose factors that would make it ethical, safe, practical, marketable, and results-oriented. Finally, I wanted the results to be lasting. The paragraphs that follow explain how the WHY Program meets each of these criteria. I ask that you follow every recommendation in this chapter, in order to conduct the WHY Program in the most professional way possible.

Ethical Criteria

The WHY Program was developed to be administered by licensed or certified psychotherapists, counselors, nutritionists, physicians, pastoral counselors, mental-health personnel, or medical personnel who have obtained certification training in hypnotherapy and NLP. In conducting this program, follow the ethical and legal guidelines of your profession as well as of your certification and licensing boards and the legislative bodies in your locality. You must also have had training and instruction in the safe and ethical use of clinical hypnosis and must consistently apply what you have learned with every client, for every session.

Please note that this program is intended for individual counseling and therapy with adults and, with written parental consent, older teens (roughly age fifteen or older). It is not intended for children, although the age fifteen cutoff is somewhat arbitrary. It is not intended for groups. For more about contraindications, see chapter 3, "WHY Program Overview."

Be advised that recent U.S. federal legislation requires all medical and mental-health practitioners to inform clients in writing as to their rights to privacy and confidentiality. Client confidentiality should be observed at all times. I recommend that you have the client sign an informed consent agreement prior to engaging your services. Such an agreement informs your clients about your policies and practices, client confidentiality and privacy, your fee arrangements, and the specific requirements of the WHY Program. The informed consent agreement lays out the expectations of the client and practitioner in advance, so that both parties can avoid misunderstandings. I recommend that you keep one signed copy in the client's file and send another copy home with the client, so that the client can save it as a reference. If you have a standard form that you use, you may want to modify it for the WHY Program or add an addendum outlining the program's specific requirements. In appendix C, I have included a sample informed consent agreement, which you can adapt and modify for use in your practice or clinical setting.

The requirements of the WHY Program are that the client

- actively participates in a physician-approved dietary or nutritional program while enrolled in the WHY Program
- has undergone a recent physical examination during which a physician has advised him or her regarding appropriate weight reduction goals, nutrition and diet, and exercise
- is advised as to the proper way to use the audio recordings produced during the WHY Program (in sessions 5–8)
- has been advised about the safety and uses of clinical hypnotherapy
- has received information about your policies regarding privacy and confidentiality
- understands the fee structure of the program and pays the fee in advance.

Safety Criteria

Prior to submitting the manuscript of this book for publication, I asked Ms. Carol Epner, a registered nurse specializing in health, nutrition, and obesity to review it for the safety and appropriateness of the medical and nutritional information in it. Her feedback in this regard has proved invaluable. I believe that the WHY Program is safe if the practitioner follows the guidelines and recommendations in the next paragraphs.

First, as I have mentioned, prior to enrolling in the WHY Program the client should have a thorough medical evaluation in which he or she discusses with a physician appropriate goals for weight reduction, diet and nutrition, and exercise. For clients who have chronic obesity, I recommend that the physician do tests to rule out medical problems that contribute to weight gain (and difficulty with weight reduction). You'll find a list of such problems in chapter 3 under "Contraindications."

One type of physician who treats patients with chronic obesity is a bariatrician.[2] Bariatricians treat obesity with a comprehensive program of diet, exercise, lifestyle changes, and, when indicated, the prescription of appetite suppressants and other appropriate medications. According to the American Society of Bariatric Physicians (2005),

While any licensed physician can offer a medical weight loss program to patients, Bariatric Physicians have been exposed, through an extensive continuing medical education program, to specialized knowledge, tools, and techniques to enable them to design specialized medical weight loss programs tailored to the needs of individual patients and modify the programs, if needed, as the treatment progresses. … A physician-supervised medical weight loss program may be the safest and wisest way to lose weight and maintain the loss. Overweight and obesity are frequently accompanied by other medical conditions, such as type 2 diabetes, hypertension, cancer, and others. A Bariatric Physician is trained to detect and treat these conditions, which might go undetected and untreated in a non-medical weight loss program.

Second, in order to participate in the WHY Program, clients must be enrolled and actively participating in a medically approved nutrition/diet program or plan that meets individual nutritional and dietary needs based on their current health and medical history. Whatever nutritional plan or program my clients choose, I advise them to check first with their physician or a nutrition specialist to make sure it is appropriate and suitable. Unless you are a dietitian or nutritionist (in addition to being an NLP practitioner and hypnotherapist), you are unlikely to have sufficient expertise to advise your clients about dietary and nutritional concerns. If you venture into giving medical or nutritional advice without proper training and credentials, you could give incorrect information and run the risk of unethical practice. Your client's signature on the informed consent agreement, attesting that (a) he or she has met with a physician, and (b) is participating in a physician-approved nutrition or dietary program, is your verification that these important safety requirements have been satisfied.

Third, because the WHY Program uses hypnosis audio recordings (more about audio recording in the next two chapters), you'll want to make sure that your client receives written guidelines as to the appropriate way to use these recordings. I urge you to include the following information in your informed consent agreement or addendum (see the sample informed consent agreement in appendix C).

- Since hypnosis audio recordings usually instruct the listener to relax, close his or her eyes, and sometimes concentrate, imagine, or visualize, it is imperative to listen to them in an environment that is relatively free of distractions. The client certainly should not listen to the recordings while operating a vehicle or potentially dangerous equipment.
- The client should not listen to the recording while caring for others who may require ongoing supervision (such as small children or incapacitated adults).
- Each recording is for the client's personal use and should not be passed along to or reproduced for another person. Should this occur, you are not

responsible for the outcome, as you have no contractual agreement with any third party.

- For the same reason, the client should not reproduce the recordings for distribution or use the recordings for any commercial purpose (which would actually be a violation of copyright). The recordings are intended for the client's personal use, not for resale or reproduction.

Fourth, I advise you to approach this program with the client's internal ecology foremost in mind. Attending to the client's ecology means that you help the client establish behavioral outcomes that are consistent with his or her values, relationships, roles, responsibilities, health, and safety. This is the best way to avoid internal conflicts that undermine motivation and resolve.

For example, when you and your client establish well-written outcomes and specify the desired results, make sure that the client has set a realistic target weight and maintains healthy, realistic expectations for weight reduction. A healthy expectation is one or two pounds (approximately one kilo) per week. More than two pounds a week is not recommended because such rapid weight loss causes the body to conserve calories (energy) and actually slows the metabolism, which makes long-term weight reduction much more difficult. Additionally, if the client is not exercising regularly while reducing weight, the body sacrifices muscle rather than fat reserves.

All of this may seem to be common sense, but common sense is becoming rather uncommon, and given our litigious society, it is best to err on the side of caution. Although the purpose of this book is not to advise you about managing your professional liabilities, I strongly advise that you carry ample liability malpractice insurance and stay up-to-date about local and national legislation that affects the administrative and ethical conduct of your practice.

Practical Considerations

The WHY Program is practical in that it addresses the day-to-day dilemmas and challenges that clients who are overweight face most often. It is also practical for you, the practitioner, in that it is intended as a *model* for you to follow and adapt to your own clinical preferences and the individual needs of each client. Part II of this book presents eight sessions that serve as a blueprint for the WHY Program. If for some reason the content or methods of any sessions are not appropriate for you or your client, you'll find a general-purpose session in chapter 14 and additional interventions in part III that you can use in place of those in part II. Thus, you can follow the program as you find it in part II or you can mix and match that content with your own methods or with processes in part III.

Here is an overview of the WHY Program blueprint: The first session focuses on explaining the program, interviewing the client, clarifying expectations, taking care of administrative details, establishing workable outcomes, and getting the client's commitment. The second session uses reframing to help the client resolve internal conflicts about food. The next session teaches self-hypnosis for weight control. Self-hypnosis puts more control into the client's hands and provides a tool for accomplishing behavioral changes. The fourth session enhances stress management skills—something most individuals with weight issues need.

The next four sessions (sessions 5–8) are scripted hypnotherapy sessions, in which you record the session then give the recording to the client. You can adapt these scripts to clients' individual needs. Each session addresses a common problem in weight management: food selection (session 5), eating patterns (session 6), and motivation to exercise (session 7). The final session (8) is designed to consolidate the client's accomplishments, reinforce progress, and promote lasting change.

In addition to giving the client audio recordings, you will be giving take-home assignments from the *WHY Client Workbook*, so that clients can (a) remain mindful of their desired outcomes, (b) learn more about nutrition and weight management, (c) acquire additional problem-solving strategies, and (d) take direct action to accomplish results. You can also add your own take-home materials, if you wish. The workbook assignments are contained on the accompanying CD, so that you can easily and cost-effectively print whatever materials you need.

Marketability Considerations

To attract clients who can benefit from your services, you must offer them something of value. When it comes to hypnotherapy, clients want a program that is not only practical (i.e., addresses their daily challenges and dilemmas), but can be accomplished in a reasonable time at a reasonable price. I believe eight sessions constitutes a reasonable time frame in which to address the most common behavioral problems of obesity. In your own practice, you might find you are successful with more or fewer sessions. For those clients who want more support, you can offer additional follow-up sessions (at your usual fee) that address specific concerns.

I prefer the eight-session model because each session is designed to address an important facet of weight management. I occasionally encounter prospective clients who assume that hypnotherapy will solve significant, chronic problems in only one or two sessions and ask if I could shorten the program to meet their expectations. I rarely do so unless I can determine that the client is already successful with most aspects of weight management—already exercising regularly and already reducing weight, for example. Not everyone can afford eight sessions and some are not willing to pay for eight hours of my time, but for most people who have experience with psychotherapy, counseling, or change work, the number of sessions is within their expectations. The point of establishing a specific number of sessions is so that clients can calculate in advance how much time and money they will spend with me—and so that I can articulate exactly what I have to offer.

Emphasis on Results

No program is worthwhile, for you or your clients, unless it gets the expected results. When clients get the results they want, they may tell their friends about you. They may want to come back to you for other services. When I designed the WHY Program, I wanted a way to ensure that clients would indeed finish the program weighing less than they did when they began.

Please keep this in mind: By U.S. medical standards, obesity generally means being forty pounds (approximately eighteen kilos) or more over one's recommended weight. Obviously, if the client visits you every week, or every other week, he or she is not likely to reduce those forty (or more) pounds over the course of the eight sessions. Instead, the WHY Program helps clients make specific lifestyle changes that result in an initial weight reduction while they are in the program. After the eight sessions, they can use the methods, information, and tools you have given them to continue making progress. One client told me that the WHY Program gave her a "jump-start" on weight management. That's exactly what this program does. Clients can also come back to see you for follow-up sessions as needed (see chapter 18).

Clients will reduce in weight while on this program (I will tell you how you can be sure they do later in this chapter). Then, after the eight sessions are complete, they are expected to maintain the changes and continue dropping excess weight until they have attained a target weight. If a client wants to come back for additional follow-up or refresher sessions with you, you can arrange this—and it is a good idea. Follow-up sessions allow you to help clients over any additional challenges on the road to a healthy weight. You can also support them in the event they start to slide back into old habits.

What kind of results can you and your clients expect with the WHY Program? Every client who completes the WHY Program will reduce his or her weight by *at least sixteen pounds (eight kilos)*. How is that possible? Because of the "accountability factor," which is an element that makes the program work. This factor is important because when you hold people accountable, they produce results.

The WHY Program holds clients accountable for making progress. Here's how it works:

1. The client must pay for the entire program in advance. No pay-as-you-go, no discounts, no credit, no payment plan. Every client must pay the entire fee up-front, at the first session. From an administrative perspective, you can justify the one-time up-front payment, because the client is not purchasing billable hours from you. Instead, the client is purchasing a complete program of services, audiotapes or CDs, and reading materials.

2. There is *no refund.* Instead of offering a money-back guarantee (if the client is not satisfied) that allows for the possibility of failure, you are upping the ante. You must tell clients from the very beginning that there are no refunds. The reason is this: You want to make sure each client is totally committed to getting results—and results are only possible by completing the program. This incentive prevents people from dropping out and then asking for a refund. The "no refund" rule encourages clients to "get their money's worth" from you by carrying out the assignments, reading the materials, listening to the recordings, and completing all eight sessions. If the client doesn't complete the program, you still keep the payment. By the way, I don't place a time limit by which clients must return or forfeit the payment. My clients have a standing invitation to return to my office any time to complete the program, at no additional charge, even if I have increased my overall fees since their last session.

3. Through completing the program, every client will reduce his or her weight by at least sixteen pounds (or eight kilos), because after the fourth session, the client cannot return for each subsequent session until he or she has lost four pounds (or two kilos). Doing so usually means an interim of about two or three weeks between sessions—sometimes longer—because clients work at their own pace. Here's how the program produces a minimum weight reduction of sixteen pounds (or eight kilos):
    *   The client completes session 4 and reduces four pounds (or two kilos).
    *   The client returns, completes session 5, and reduces an additional four pounds (or two more kilos), for a total of eight pounds (or four kilos).
    *   The client returns, completes session 6, and reduces an additional four pounds (two more kilos), for a total of twelve pounds (or six kilos).
    *   The client returns, completes session 7 and reduces an additional four pounds (two more kilos), for a total of sixteen pounds (or eight kilos).
    *   The client returns for session 8, the final session, having reduced sixteen pounds (or eight kilos) in total and being well on the way to his or her target weight.

You may be wondering how you can be sure your clients have reduced by the required weight between sessions. Use an honor system. Trust is an important component of any therapeutic relationship. Let your clients know that they are responsible for reporting their weight accurately. If a client lies about the reduced poundage, that's a matter of conscience. You do not need to keep a scale in your office area, because clients can be expected to weigh themselves at home, a fitness center, or a clinic. This policy helps clients avoid the embarrassment of stepping on a scale in your presence, while simultaneously putting the onus on them to get on a scale somewhere.

If you want to keep a scale handy, that's fine. I caution you, however, that many clients are mortified about weighing themselves in front of another person, because they feel a great deal of shame attached to their weight. If you have a scale in your office, be very sensitive to clients' feelings and never convey dismay, pity, or disapproval.

The accountability factor is an important element in the program's efficacy. Remember, it consists of three components:

1. The client pays the full fee up-front.
2. There are no refunds.
3. After the fourth session, the client must reduce four pounds (two kilos) in order to return for each subsequent session, reducing his or her weight by at least sixteen pounds (eight kilos) by the final session.

The accountability factor is that simple, and it works as an incentive to weight reduction. Moreover, it allows the client to advance through the program on the basis of small, incremental successes, and to see actual results. Make certain your clients understand the three stipulations in advance of the first session, and get their agreement in writing. Your informed consent agreement should cover these three points.

Clients can work through the program at their own pace and on their own schedule. I do not impose time frames for completing the program or dropping weight. I leave that up to my clients. Some of my clients have completed the program in three or four months; others have taken a year. I also allow clients to put any remaining WHY Program sessions "on hold" in order to insert additional counseling sessions around other issues that arise while they are enrolled in the program. (Clients pay for these sessions separately.) Matty (not her real name), for example, had completed six sessions in the program when her fiancé broke off their engagement. She was understandably upset. We put the seventh and eighth sessions "on hold" and spent an additional two sessions processing her feelings about the breakup. Then, when she was ready, we went back and finished the seventh and eighth sessions of the WHY Program.

Lasting Results

Clients frequently ask, "Will the results last?" Obviously, no practitioner can make such a guarantee, because it's impossible to predict what circumstances will befall clients or what decisions they will make over the remainder of a lifetime. Nevertheless, it is understandable that clients, in particular those who are overweight, would want reassurances of lasting results. Most clients come to you having struggled with their weight for years, slimming down and then regaining those pounds many times over. Some of my clients have told me hypnotherapy is their "last resort."

For these reasons, the WHY Program was designed to give lasting results, by putting the tools and methods into the client's hands. Having completed the program, your client will know self-hypnosis, have a method for stress management, and have four customized hypnotherapy audiotapes or CDs, all to provide the skills and tools needed to sustain change over time. In this sense, the WHY Program encourages the client to be self-reliant in weight management. In eight sessions, he or she has acquired methods, information, and tools that will last, we hope, for a lifetime.

Additionally, you can continue to work with any client beyond the eight sessions. In this book you'll find a "bonus" session, ideas for coaching clients who are stuck, recommendations for follow-up sessions, and additional NLP patterns for working with overeating. For some clients, those first sixteen pounds (eight kilos) will give them the momentum for ongoing success, and the first eight sessions will give them the confidence to return for additional support when they hit rough spots.

Chapter 3

WHY Program Overview

The WHY Program assists clients with the psychological and motivational aspects of weight reduction. Its purpose is to alleviate compulsive eating and enhance the motivation to exercise and reduce weight. The program focuses solely on these aspects of weight reduction, and on alleviating the client's *current* behaviors that are the source of overeating and obesity. Other presenting problems—such as depression and anxiety, family psychodynamics, self-esteem, grief and loss, post traumatic stress disorder, other addictions, or problematic childhood issues—should be addressed outside of this eight-session program, in additional therapy sessions. If you are not qualified to address these types of issues with your weight reduction clients, refer them to a colleague who is qualified and concentrate your efforts on helping them stay motivated to reduce weight.

The WHY Program was developed through clinical experience with actual clients, a review of clinical research studies on hypnotherapy and weight control, and consultation with numerous colleagues and a registered nurse practitioner who specializes in the development of health and nutrition programs. It is a solution-oriented, brief psychotherapy approach that focuses on the "here and now" of current behaviors related to food, eating habits, coping skills, and physical exercise. It also allows the client to work at an individual pace.

Program Outline

As I stated in the previous chapter, I am presenting the WHY Program to you in the format I most often use. Consider the eight-session program, as detailed in part II, a model that you can adapt for your own clientele. I don't promote a cookie-cutter approach, and I do expect that each practitioner who reads this book will develop useful and creative variations on the model I present. Some of you might want to decrease or increase the number of sessions. Some of you might want to vary the scripts, or even substitute scripts of your own choosing. Some of you might want to substitute the NLP patterns in chapter 16 for one or more of the scripted hypnotherapy sessions.

In my version of the WHY Program, the first four sessions draw from NLP and the last four draw from Ericksonian hypnosis (although there is certainly overlap in both approaches, since NLP was derived from Ericksonian hypnosis). I schedule these sessions for 60 minutes. Depending on the pace at which you work, you might want to schedule 75-minute, or perhaps even 90-minute, sessions—you be the judge of what will work best for you. (Remember: You'll be making audio recordings of the hypnotherapy scripts in sessions 5 through 8, so these need to be short enough to fit on a CD or audio cassette.) The following outline gives an overview of the sessions as they appear in this book.

1. Intake Interview and Introduction to the WHY Program
2. Reframing Compulsive Eating
3. Training in Self-Hypnosis
4. Stopping Emotional Eating with Stress Management
5. Making Sensible Food Choices
6. Creating an Intelligent Relationship with Food
7. Boosting Motivation to Exercise
8. Pulling It All Together for Lasting Results

Chapters 6 through 13 each cover one session in detail, and chapter 14 contains a "bonus session." Although each session addresses a separate aspect of weight management, you can expect some overlap in session content. Each chapter contains the following information: (a) purpose, (b) step-by-step procedures, (c) scripts that accompany the procedures, (d) client take-home assignments (these are in the *Client Workbook* on the accompanying CD), and (e) checklist and notes.

The client materials are the same ones I use in my practice. Some assignments have been adapted or excerpted from the book *Healthy Habits*. Each assignment is titled to indicate the session it accompanies. If you have relevant materials of your own, feel free to give those to your clients also.

You may photocopy the appropriate "Practitioner Checklist and Notes," fill it out during the session, and place it in the client's file. The "Checklist" section is a convenient way of making sure you have covered all the activities for the session. It also provides a record of each session and a quick reference to remember which sessions you have completed with a particular client. Use the "Notes" section to write down important things to remember about the client: personality traits, feedback, successes, and client-specific concerns. These notes will help you customize the hypnotherapy scripts for each client, and will be especially helpful in assembling suggestions for the last hypnotherapy script in session 8.

The Scripts

Chapters 7 through 9 (sessions 2 through 4) each contain a sample script that takes the client through the Six-Step Reframe, self-hypnosis training, and anchoring a resourceful state. In delivering these scripts, you can use either a conversational or a hypnotic voice, as you deem appropriate. My hypnotic voice, for example, is a bit slower and more rhythmical than my usual conversational voice. I rarely explicitly announce to my client that I'm switching from one voice to the other. I usually segue from one to the other with a "linking" phrase such as, "And now as you are thinking about what we were discussing, you might consider... ."

Chapters 10 through 13 contain hypnotherapy scripts for sessions 5 through 8. Each script follows this general structure.

Induction and Reassurances

Each script begins with an *induction,* to help the client relax and focus concentration, and to establish the purpose and tone of the hypnotherapy session. Following the induction and throughout the script, you may want to add your own deepening suggestions, depending on your style and the client's comfort level and expectations.

The induction includes *reassurances.* The primary purpose of the reassurances is to address the concerns of clients who may be somewhat apprehensive or unfamiliar with hypnosis. Some people experiencing hypnosis for the first time worry that they may be immobilized during trance, unable to respond to emergencies, or that the therapist may inadvertently give them a suggestion that brings dire consequences.

The reassurances are intended to allay such fears and help the client have a comfortable, satisfying trance experience. The second purpose of reassurances is to limit your liability in case the client may one day engage in some inappropriate or risky behavior and then attribute the behavior to something heard in a hypnotherapy session. For this reason, I recommend that you record the reassurances on every audiotape (even though it may seem gratuitous to do so). The reassurances are these (note that ellipses represent pauses):

> While you are relaxing now, here are some things to remember, for your comfort, safety, and satisfaction with this hypnosis experience. No matter how deeply relaxed you feel, you are free to move about to become even more comfortable. You can open your eyes and end this process at any time you desire and for any reason you desire. While you are listening to this tape, should anything occur that requires your immediate attention, you will instantly return to full alertness, open your eyes, move about, and attend to the matter without delay.
>
> No matter ... *how deeply ... relaxed you are, you are free to accept or reject anything I say.* If I say something that isn't helpful or relevant ... your mind will automatically dismiss it and ignore it. It will have no negative effect whatsoever. ... To the same extent, when I say *suggestions that are useful and helpful, then I trust ... your inner mind will absorb these ideas and recommendations ... integrating them with your beliefs and values, altering your perceptions and understandings, so that ... desirable changes are becoming evident ... in your thinking, feel-*

23

ing, and acting ... in ways that are healthy and positive . . so that in the days and weeks to follow ... you are experiencing benefits and improvements ... physically ... mentally ... and emotionally.

Change Work

The "Change Work" section in each script introduces ideas, analogies, metaphors, NLP patterns, and direct suggestions for change. This is where the main work of the script takes place.

Posthypnotic Suggestions and Future Rehearsal

The posthypnotic suggestions and future rehearsal vary for each script. This section is the part of the script that tells the client to plan and expect that the changes are taking place and the desired results are forthcoming.

Reinforcement

The "Reinforcement" section encourages the client to listen to the recording multiple times, sets an expectation of positive results, and affirms his or her progress. It reads as follows:

> I recommend that each time you listen to this recording, the positive suggestions be more effective and powerful ... enhancing your progress. The changes in your thought patterns and behaviors ... more productive and satisfying.

Ending and Reorientation

Each script concludes with an ending and reorientation section, which allows clients the option of drifting into sleep (if they are listening to the recording at night in bed, just before sleep) or of regaining alertness and returning to the day's activities. I use this dual ending because I find that clients often don't have time to listen to the recordings during their daily routine, and many prefer to listen to the recordings as a way to relax just before falling asleep at night. I recommend that clients who listen to the recordings while drifting into sleep use an audio cassette or CD player with an automatic shutoff for convenience. Another solution for busy clients is to set the morning alarm about thirty or forty minutes earlier, turn on the tape or CD player, and listen to the recording in bed, while still somewhat relaxed and drowsy. The ending and reorientation is as follows:

If you are listening to this recording at night in bed ... and you wish to go on to sleep ... you can simply keep on relaxing ... moving into a healthy, restorative sleep. ... I wish you lovely dreams that amplify all positive suggestions ... and I suggest that you will wake up refreshed in the morning. If you wish to drift into sleep, just ignore the following instructions. [Pause about ten seconds before continuing.]

On the other hand, if you are listening to this recording during the day and wish to return to the day's activities, [Pick up the tempo of your voice here.] give me your attention because now it's time to become fully alert again. Feel yourself become more alert, coming up now, feeling more energized, ready to return to conscious, wakeful awareness, fully alert now, eyes open, feeling fine. [When doing this with the client in your office, make sure he or she is fully alert at this time.]

Even though it is repetitive, I have included the "Reassurances," "Reinforcement," and "Ending and Reorientation" sections in every hypnotherapy script in part II, to save you the inconvenience of having to flip pages back and forth when recording. I encourage you to adapt the wording of each script to your own ways of working with clients, and to the needs and sensitivities of each client.

You certainly do not have to memorize the scripts in this book. I see nothing wrong with reading to the client directly from the book. I have done this with clients, explaining that I sometimes read scripts so that I can have a good idea of what I want to say while they are in trance, and because I have selected specific wording and suggestions that I think will address their needs. I've never had a client question or object to my reading from a script.

The scripts are intended to address the physical, emotional, and cognitive components of change. Each script focuses on a central purpose and theme. The central purpose of the script for session 5 is to select nutritious food, and the theme is to make distinctions, notice differences, and be choosy. The central purpose of the script for session 6 is to eat when hungry and stop eating when full, and the theme is self-awareness and paying attention to the body's messages. The central purpose of the script for session 7 is exercise and the theme is motivation. The central purpose of session 8 is to reinforce and review what the client has learned and accomplished, and the theme is self-acceptance, self-affirmation, and lasting results.

The scripts are inspired by the work of the late Dr. Milton H. Erickson and others who have followed in his footsteps, most notably Kay Thompson (now deceased), Roger P. Allen, Richard Bandler, John Grinder, L. Michael Hall, Bob Bodenhamer, and John Burton. You will find that the scripts contain direct and indirect suggestions, analogies, affirmations, imagery, associations, and metaphor. In the hypnotic language patterns you may encounter Sleight of Mouth Patterns, alliteration, unexpected shifts in verb tenses, homonyms and double entendres, incomplete sentences, run-on sentences, statements about cause-and-effect, rhymes, repetition, generalizations, attribution, ambiguity, and so forth, all selected to facilitate the trance experience and stimulate new thinking by the client. The general style is intended to be supportive, permissive, and non-authoritarian.

Often in the scripts you will encounter *italic type*. The italics highlight what most hypnotherapists refer to as embedded suggestions—direct suggestions to the client, marked out for the subconscious mind by a change in tone of voice. Whereas your conversational voice speaks to the conscious mind, your deeper, hypnotic voice speaks to the subconscious. When you encounter the italics, I recommend you lower your voice as a way of marking these suggestions for the client's subconscious awareness.

You will also frequently encounter ellipses (…) in the scripts, as an indication to pause briefly while reading. In general, you should read the scripts at a slow, steady pace, matching your breathing to your client's breathing (when it is comfortable for you to do so), and begin speaking on the exhale. In this way, you will develop a rhythmic way of speaking to the client that enhances relaxation and rapport.

Finally, the scripts also contain instructions to you, the practitioner, in parentheses and regular type (not italic). These instructions are not to be read to the client.

Additional Tips on Language

You will obviously want to modify the wording of the scripts for individual clients' needs and sensitivities. For example, I once had a client who did not like to hear the word "relax." When she was a child, an older, bigger, male family member would tease her by holding her tightly in a restraining manner. When she became frightened and tried to break away, he would laugh and tell her to relax. Thus, the word "relax" brought up some distressing memories for her. When I worked with this client, I substituted the words "find comfort" for "relax." A few people have negative associations with other words commonly used in hypnotherapy, such as "deep" or "floating" or "drifting." During your initial interview, ask the client about any such negative associations, and then use your judgment accordingly when reading and adapting the scripts.

Now I want to tell you about some of the language I use in describing this program to clients and prospective clients. As a practitioner, you've no doubt had training in the importance of selecting the right words to enhance rapport, create positive associations, and provide solution-oriented influences. The following are some guidelines for the best ways I've found to talk to clients about the WHY Program.

You will notice that the scripts do not contain the word "diet," and in general when I talk to clients about nutrition and meal planning, I avoid the word "diet." Most of my clients have had so many failures with diets that the word has negative connotations. Did you ever notice that the word "diet" contains the word "die?" I've often wondered if people make an unconscious association between the word "diet" and death, and that's why so many people fail at dieting. People usually complete (or give up on) whatever diet they have been on, and then return to their old habits and regain the weight they've lost.

Moreover, many people associate diets with starvation and deprivation. Diets are formulaic, and many do not teach people how to make the lifestyle and attitudinal changes that lead to lasting results. I use "dietary plan," "nutritional program," or "food plan" to avoid the negative associations with the word "diet" and to communicate to clients that they are pursuing not just weight reduction but a program that truly addresses their nutritional requirements. I remind them that the program or plan they choose should be approved by their physician, dietitian, or nutritionist. Instead of talking about "being on a diet" or "sticking to your diet," I speak to clients about "having an intelligent relationship with food" and "sensible eating" and "making healthful food choices."

I also avoid the term "weight loss" because "loss" is a word associated with sadness and mourning. Moreover, if you "lose" something, where did you put it? If you "lose" something, the implication is that you should find it or get it back. In speaking to clients about the WHY Program I use the terms "weight management" or "weight control" or "weight reduction" instead of "weight loss." I use phrases such as "shed excess pounds" or "melt away that fat" instead of "lose weight."

I do not tell clients that they will become "thin," "slender," or "slim" as a result of the WHY Program. Most obese people cannot imagine or believe that they will ever be thin or slender or slim. Instead, I use phrases such as "reach your target weight," "achieve a healthy weight," "have your favorite weight," or "have the weight you choose." Ask your clients what words they prefer when they describe the result they want.

In talking about hypnosis and the mind, I refer to the "conscious mind" and the "subconscious mind." I explain that the conscious mind is generally defined as that part of the mind that is logical, analytical, and capable of reason. I then explain that there are many definitions of the subconscious mind, and I usually just refer to it as that part of the mind that becomes more suggestible and accessible during hypnosis. If you prefer another definition, then use the one you prefer.

I am aware that there are many terms for the subconscious mind. Some practitioners, following the tradition of Dr. Milton H. Erickson, prefer to use "unconscious mind," as opposed to "subconscious mind." Personally, I prefer "subconscious" because, to me, "unconscious" implies lack of awareness or being "knocked out." I believe that people always retain awareness at some level, even in deep trance. There are also several euphemisms for the subconscious mind such as "inner mind," "inner wisdom," or "intuition." If you prefer any of these terms, simply substitute it whenever you encounter "subconscious mind" in the scripts throughout this manual.

Many clients are concerned about hypnotherapy being some kind of mind control. I counter this concern with an NLP Sleight of Mouth Pattern. I ask them how much control they have over their eating habits and their weight. They usually answer "very little." I then explain that they are already obviously "out of control" in this regard, and the point of hypnosis is to put them back in control. I convey to each client that therapy is a mutual endeavor, in which we work together as a team toward a mutually agreed on outcome. During hypnosis sessions, I also give clients reassurances that I have no intention of controlling their thoughts—only of motivating them to achieve their desired outcomes. Recall that the hypnotherapy scripts contain reassurances, to repeatedly assure clients that they are not losing control.

Last, I avoid exaggerated claims, hype, wild promises, and guarantees of success, as I consider these to be unethical. I convey to my clients that I am a practitioner offering a service. I am happy to tell them about my credentials, but I am not in business to impress them with my knowledge or expertise. I believe that the client, not the practitioner, is the "star of the show." I am not interested in making hypnotherapy seem magical or mystical; instead, I want my clients to understand that trance is a normal, natural human state that occurs routinely throughout each day. I say nothing to imply that the WHY Program is easy or effortless. Weight reduction is *not* easy—it requires sustained action and determination over time. I give my clients credit for their successes and applaud their progress—they deserve it.

Ending Each Session

When you have finished recording the script, ask your client to sit quietly and mentally review the session for any concerns or questions. You might even want your client to close his or her eyes and revisit the trance briefly for this purpose. This step will help the client to surface any ecological concerns and address them on the spot.

I am well aware that some hypnotherapy books and trainers advise against this step in order to promote posthypnotic amnesia for the session, so that the client's subconscious mind will more easily incorporate the hypnotic suggestions, without the interference of cognitive analysis. I disagree with that position, because unexpressed and unaddressed ecological concerns may lead to complications for the client.

Would you like an example? Here is a cautionary tale that I am telling on myself. I once had a client who told me he not only wanted to stop smoking, he wanted to completely forget that he ever was a smoker. During the hypnosis session, I suggested to him, "It will be as though you have never smoked." Nothing wrong with that—or so I thought! The next day I received an e-mail from the man's wife, saying that she was very worried about him. Each time she mentioned anything to him about smoking, he angrily insisted to her that he had never smoked in his life! He was saying the same thing to friends and coworkers, much to their confusion. He couldn't figure out why all these people were saying these ridiculous things to him, and he wished they would stop it.

I phoned the man on the pretext of verifying his next appointment. He said he remembered me and, yes, he remembered our next appointment. His only problem, he said, was that he couldn't remember *why* he had come to see me in the first place, or why he would be coming back to see me again the following week! When I reminded him that he had come to see me for smoking cessation, he was confused, thinking I was playing a joke on him. It took me a while to convince him that he really had been a smoker only days before.

It was good for this man to stop smoking, but it was hurtful to his relationships for him to forget that he had ever smoked! After my conversation with the client, I called a trusted colleague and mentor, Ron Klein, director of the American Hypnosis Training Academy in Silver Spring, Maryland, for supervision.[3] I asked him where I had gone wrong with that client. Ron reviewed the session with me and asked if I had conducted an ecological check with the client at the end of it.

I said yes, I had briefly and perfunctorily asked the client if he felt okay or had any questions or concerns. "But did you allow him to re-access the trance experience?" Ron asked. Well, no, I hadn't. Then Ron said to me, "A trance is a state-dependent learning experience. If the client encounters anything during the trance that poses a concern, he will not remember it when the trance is over. He has to get back into the trance in order to recall whatever might be a source of concern." Lesson learned, and now I pass it along to you.

Rationale for Recording the Sessions

The rationale for recording the hypnotherapy scripts (in sessions 5 through 8) is that listening to the recordings gives the client an opportunity to re-experience the hypnotherapy sessions numerous times. It is generally accepted in the field of psychology that clients are more likely to obtain the best results through repeated exposure to hypnotherapy suggestions, and clients become more adept with trance work through repetition and practice.

Each recording should be approximately twenty-five to forty minutes in length, so plan your additional session tasks accordingly. Each script should fit on one side of a ninety-minute audiotape or on a CD-R (which normally holds fifty to eighty minutes of audio content). Record the hypnotherapy script as you read it with the client present in your office. Doing so allows you to calibrate your pace and wording to the client's breathing, facial expressions, and other responses during the recording process.

For example, if you say something and the client smiles, you might ad lib, "Thinking in this way brings a smile to your face." If the client seems to frown, you might say, "And you might feel a certain way about that information." Of course, if the client seems distressed during the process, it is best to stop recording, bring the client to alertness, find out what is troubling him or her, and respond accordingly.

Before recording, discuss the purpose of the session and preview the issues that will be addressed and the types of suggestions you'll be making. Ask whether the client would like to hear anything in particular during hypnosis, so that you can customize the script to him or her. For example, when working with one client for smoking cessation, I asked if there was anything in particular he wanted to hear on the tape that would help him. He said, "Yes. Remind me that I have prayed to Jesus to help me make this change, and he is helping me now." I added that sentence to the script, and the client was very happy with it.

By the end of the program, the client will have four scripts recorded on either audiotapes or CDs. It is up to you and your client whether you establish a specific listening schedule. I find a fixed schedule usually does not work well, because clients get busy and forget, and then feel that they have failed the assignment. I simply recommend that clients listen to the tapes as often as needed to maintain their progress—which puts the decision in their hands. If anyone wants my advice as to frequency, I say listening to a tape two or three times a week should be sufficient for most people.

Contraindications (Screening Clients)

The WHY Program accommodates the needs of most individuals who are overweight or obese. It is not a panacea for every client who walks through your door for weight reduction, however. Some people have far more significant problems to solve than a flabby physique. If you are careful and selective in your choice of candidates for the WHY Program, you do yourself and your clientele a favor, and develop a good success rate in the process. Therefore, I offer the following cautions and contraindications for the WHY Program, and frankly, for any other cognitive-behavioral weight reduction program.

As mentioned in chapter 2, your client should have a thorough medical exam to rule out any previously undetected medical issues that may be contributing to weight gain or preventing weight reduction. A number of medical problems contribute to weight gain or make weight reduction more difficult. If the medical condition can be controlled or treated sufficiently to allow full participation in and benefit from the WHY Program, and if the client continues to be under medical supervision for the duration of the program, you may decide to enroll the person at your discretion. A client with any of the following problems should be under a physician's care to treat these problems:

- hormonal imbalances (women only): symptoms include fatigue, cravings for sweets, weight gain, depression, premenstrual syndrome, mood swings, insomnia, anxiety, joint pain, hair loss, and irregular menstruation
- hypothyroidism (a malfunction of the thyroid gland): symptoms include fatigue, depression, and weight gain
- metabolic syndrome (a condition in which the body cannot use insulin efficiently): the symptoms are obesity and high blood pressure. This condition poses an elevated risk for cardiovascular disease
- hyper-insulinemia (an endocrine disorder affecting the body's ability to control blood sugar; a forerunner of type 2 diabetes). The symptoms are fatigue, obesity or problems reducing weight, and mood swings
- insulin-dependent diabetes (type 1 diabetes, in which the pancreas produces too little insulin to regulate blood sugar, altering the metabolism of fats, proteins, and sugars): symptoms include fatigue, abdominal pain, increased urination, thirst, and absence of menstruation
- an active malignancy (cancerous cells)
- cardiac disease (malfunction of the heart and clogging of arteries)
- kidney disease
- recent surgery
- pregnancy or lactation (dieting during this time can endanger the health of the fetus or infant)
- anorexia or bulimia

- polycystic ovarian syndrome (women only): symptoms include enlarged ovaries with small cysts, causing a disruption in hormonal cycles, infertility, insulin resistance, obesity, and a masculine appearance.

Practitioners should exercise clinical judgment and caution when implementing the WHY Program with individuals who are elderly, have physical disabilities, or have a history of anorexia or bulimia. Consulting with the client's primary care physician is wise before conducting any weight reduction program with these types of individuals.

The WHY Program is also contraindicated for clients who are in the midst of a major life crisis, since they should be concentrating their energies on more pressing concerns than weight reduction. It is contraindicated for clients who are actively abusing alcohol, illegal drugs, or prescription drugs, because the impairments and complications of these addictions may interfere with the ability to participate fully and successfully in the program. For the same reasons, the program is contraindicated for individuals with active psychotic disorders or moderate to profound mental retardation or dementia. The WHY Program is not intended for group therapy, children, or individuals who are within twelve pounds (five kilos) of their target weight.

This program may benefit teenagers, provided they are self-motivated and have full parental permission, support, and supervision (and you have written parental consent). The WHY Program is contraindicated for teens who are presenting with other issues such as oppositional behavior, acting out, delinquency, truancy, drug and alcohol use, sexuality concerns, or depression, as these issues are far more urgent than weight concerns, and the associated stresses will most likely interfere with their ability to participate fully and successfully in a weight reduction program.

The WHY Program is not recommended for individuals who maintain unrealistic expectations as to their desired weight and the extent to which clinical interventions can help them, or for those who do not wish to comply with program requirements (i.e., consult a physician, pay the full fee, get on a nutritional plan, choose a form of exercise, and reduce weight by four pounds, or two kilos, after each of sessions 4 through 7).

Maintain Your Adaptability

The content, methods, and wording of the eight sessions in this program will not be ideally suited to the needs of every client, so you will want to maintain some creative adaptability, using the program outline as a framework. Vary the WHY Program in accordance with each client's needs and your own clinical judgment. Here are some variations I have used in my practice:

One of my clients had just completed the fourth session when her brother passed on. She was overcome with grief. We put her remaining sessions on hold and spent the next month in grief counseling, as she worked through the loss. At the end of the month, she resumed the program.

Another client completed the fifth session of the program and then announced, to my surprise, that she wanted to take an indefinite hiatus. I wrongly assumed she would drop out. Instead, she continued to call me on a monthly basis with reports of steady weight reduction. At the end of six months, she had reduced her weight by forty pounds (approximately eighteen kilos) and had reached her target weight. Since she still had three more program sessions, I told her she could use those sessions to address any topics she wanted. We spent those remaining sessions on stress management, self-esteem, and belief change.

Another client asked me to reverse the order of the fourth and fifth sessions (on stress management and healthy food choices, respectively). Why? Because following the fourth session, she was going away on a two-week vacation. She was certain she would have little stress during her vacation but many temptations to eat unhealthy, fattening foods. The switch made perfect sense.

When clients have completed the eight sessions, you might want to offer "refresher," "follow-up," or "maintenance" sessions to address other relevant issues not covered in the program (such as self-esteem or self-confidence) or new, unanticipated, or feared dilemmas that arise with weight reduction (such as how to accommodate a new body image or a more attractive appearance). See chapter 18 "Suggestions for Follow-up Sessions." You could even conduct a weight-maintenance counseling or coaching group with clients who have completed the WHY Program.

Chapter 4

Your Preparation

Now that you have an overview of the WHY Program, you will want to make sure you have enough preparatory information to implement the program smoothly. That is the purpose of this chapter. First, I review the clinical skills that pertain to the program and what you should know about weight management. The remainder of the chapter contains practical advice and instructions about weight reduction resources, making the audio recordings, setting your fee, and your own "moment of truth" about weight.

Clinical Skills

The skills you need to conduct the WHY Program are those you are probably already using in your practice and ones you have most likely encountered in your professional training. It takes a lot more than just reading scripts to perform quality hypnotherapy. To conduct the WHY Program, you'll benefit from the skills necessary to accomplish the following activities:

* Establish rapport with the client.
* Conduct an intake interview.
* Explain what hypnotherapy and NLP are, and answer the client's questions knowledgeably.
* Calibrate behavioral indications of internal states.
* Help the client arrive at well-formed outcomes.
* Perform tests of hypnotizability.
* Train the client in self-hypnosis.
* Apply hypnotic methods: induction, deepening, guided visualization, future rehearsal, metaphor, hypnotic suggestion, and reorientation.
* Demonstrate familiarity with hypnotic language patterns.
* Perform the Six-Step Reframe.
* Guide the client in accessing and anchoring a resourceful state.
* Elicit the client's current strategies and teach new strategies.
* Work with a client's values and Meta-Programs.
* Use Sleight of Mouth Patterns conversationally.
* Help clients assess their ecological considerations.

At first glance, this list might seem a tall order. A closer examination reveals however that the majority of these skills are taught in most beginning-level NLP practitioner programs. It is not the purpose of this book to offer a primer on these skills (although some NLP procedures are outlined briefly in the text). If you are unfamiliar with any of these skills or vocabulary, I recommend the following steps to increase your competency:

1. Take or repeat a training program for certified NLP practitioners.
2. Consult one of the many excellent NLP texts that cover these skills. I recommend *The User's Manual for the Brain*, volumes 1 and 2 (1999b, 2003), by Hall and Bodenhamer and *The Encyclopedia of Systemic NLP and NLP New Coding* (2000), by Dilts and DeLozier.
3. Obtain peer supervision from a colleague who is certified in NLP and familiar with the listed skills.
4. Establish or participate in an NLP/hypnotherapy study/discussion group in which practitioners meet periodically to exchange professional information and provide peer evaluation and feedback. If you can't find one, start your own.

What You Should Know about Weight Management

You should have some basic knowledge about weight management, such as what is an appropriate weight for a given individual. The U.S. Department of Health and Human Services and the World Health Organization establish adult weight guidelines based on body mass index (BMI). To calculate BMI in English (or imperial) units, divide weight in pounds by height in inches squared (lb/in^2). Then multiply by 703. In metric units BMI is determined by dividing weight in kilograms by height in meters squared (kg/m^2). A BMI of 19 to 25 is considered a healthy range. A BMI of 26 to 30 is considered moderately overweight. A BMI of 31 to 35 indicates obesity, and a BMI of 36 to 40 indicates severe obesity. An individual with a BMI of more than 40 is considered morbidly obese.[4]

Don't expect every client to strive for an ideal weight within a BMI range of 19 to 25, at least not initially. Many would be happy with just reducing their girth by twenty or thirty pounds (approximately ten or fifteen kilograms), and most physicians will agree that any weight reduction at all is healthy. Let your clients set their own weight reduction goals under guidance from a physician.

Second question: What is a calorie, and what do calories have to do with weight control? A calorie is a unit of energy supplied by food. The human body needs a minimum number of calories each day just to sustain normal functioning. Table 1 overleaf shows recommended caloric intakes for women and men, based on general activity level.

People who are overweight take in more calories than their bodies need, and the body converts the unused calories into fat. What is the mechanism of weight reduction? Simple: Burn more calories than are consumed. That means in order to lose weight one must reduce caloric intake or increase calorie-burning activity or both. How many calories must one burn to accomplish one pound in weight reduction? A whopping 3,500 calories! (One kilo in weight reduction takes approximately 7,700 calories!) I am amazed at how few of my weight reduction clients know this, even though most of them have been dieting for years.

To slim down by one pound (or approximately a half kilo) in seven days, an individual would have to lower calorie intake by 500 calories a day or increase physical activity sufficiently to burn off 500 calories a day (or, more likely, a combination of both). The number of calories burned depends on the type of activity (Bannister and Brown 1968; Passmore and Dumin 1955). The approximate amount of various sustained activities needed to burn approximately 500 calories would be as follows:

- 30 minutes of walking up stairs or skiing on a skiing machine
- 60 minutes of jogging, aerobic dancing, skipping rope, tennis, or bicycling
- 120 minutes of swimming, horseback riding, dancing, badminton, or volleyball
- 150 minutes of walking, housework, or yard work

Exercise is a must because it builds muscle, burns calories, and increases metabolism. Although burning off 500 calories a day from increased activity and reduced food intake is doable, such a regimen is too extreme for most individuals. If the 500-calorie reduction comes only from reducing food, the lower calorie intake may trigger the body's energy-conservation response, which slows the metabolism. The body gets the idea that it may starve and lowers metabolism to conserve energy. A reduction of 250 calories a day is less likely to trigger the energy-conservation response. At a calorie-reduction and burn rate of 250 calories a day, an individual could drop one pound in two weeks. Even at this rate, some individuals may feel fatigue or experience moodiness, as a physiological effect of decreased caloric intake. Advise your client to set small, conservative weight reduction goals. Naturally, metabolic rates vary, and some individuals have a higher metabolism than others, burning calories more efficiently.

Recent studies show a strong correlation between inadequate sleep and obesity (Gangwisch and Heymsfield 2004). A team of researchers at Stanford University (Mignot et al. 2004) found that insufficient sleep adversely affects hormone levels associated with activity and appetite. At the University of Bristol, Taheri (2004) found that inadequate sleep lowers metabolism and causes weight gain. Ask your clients about their sleep patterns and encourage them to get a full eight hours of sleep each night. If they have trouble sleeping, set aside an extra session for addressing the problem (with relaxation training, for example) or refer them to a physician for an evaluation (or both).

Table 1. Daily caloric needs based on general activity level[5]

General Activity Level	Women	Men
Sedentary: sitting most of day, with little physical activity.	Multiply body weight (in pounds) by 14 calories. For kilos, multiply by 31 calories.	Multiply body weight (in pounds) by 15 calories. For kilos, multiply by 33 calories.
Light activity: standing most of the day.	Multiply body weight (in pounds) by 15 calories. For kilos, multiply by 35 calories.	Multiply body weight (in pounds) by 16 calories. For kilos, multiply by 35 calories.
Moderate activity: daily activity includes walking, gardening, and housework.	Multiply body weight (in pounds) by 16 calories. For kilos, multiply by 40 calories.	Multiply body weight (in pounds) by 17 calories. For kilos, multiply by 47 calories.
High activity: dancing, skating, tennis, jogging, aerobics, or manual labor such as construction work or farmwork.	Multiply body weight (in pounds) by 17 calories. For kilos, multiply by 48 calories.	Multiply body weight (in pounds) by 19 calories. For kilos, multiply by 42 calories.
	Pregnant women: add 300 calories per day.	
	Lactating women: add 500 calories per day.	
	Women over 50: subtract 250 calories per day. (Reduced estrogen decreases metabolism.)	

Source: American Cancer Society: "Calculate Your Daily Needs," Available online at <www.cancer.org/docroot/PED/content/PED61xCalorieCalculator.asp?sitearea=&level=>. These numbers may vary slightly according to the source one consults. Individual calorie needs may also vary from those recommended here.

This is the least you should know. I recommend you read some reputable books and check out web sites on healthful eating and exercise so that you can acquire sufficient knowledge to understand your clients' needs and goals and answer their concerns about balanced nutrition, calories, weight reduction, and exercise.

Familiarize Yourself with Resources

Familiarize yourself with weight reduction clinics and health facilities in your area, such as Weight Watchers, Jenny Craig, health spas, and fitness clubs. Learn about the leading weight reduction and exercise programs offered on television via the home-shopping channels and infomercials. Know something about the latest diet fads, popular diet books, medications, and over-the-counter weight-loss products.

You don't have to be an expert on these facilities, programs, diets, and pills, but you should know enough about them to recognize which ones might prove unsafe or ineffective for your clients. *Do not* promote any weight-reducing drug, over-the-counter-pill, or supplement because in the long run many such substances have proven to be ineffective or unsafe. You limit your risk of liability by telling your client to consult with a physician or nutritionist about so-called weight-loss aids.

I recommend that you *not* promote any particular diet or diet program, because studies show conclusively that diets simply do not work. Only 5 percent of people actually reach and maintain their target weight regardless of what diet plan they follow—or whether they follow a diet plan at all. Commercial diet plans, if used alone, with no other interventions, fail for 95 percent of the people who use them to manage their weight. Reducing fat intake, getting routine exercise, and learning to eat in response to the body's own sensations of hunger and satiety are far more effective for weight reduction than are diets alone (Fraser 1997). Advise your clients to get a physician's approval before investing in any diet, over-the-counter drug, or weight-loss product, meal plan, or exercise regimen. Get to know a few well-qualified nutritionists in your area and consult with them about the efficacy of local weight reduction facilities, diets, drugs, weight-loss products, and diet books and tapes. Regularly review reputable health columns, web sites, and newsletters concerning weight management to stay up-to-date.

Believe me, your clients are checking out all these weight reduction methods and may want to talk to you about them. You will have more credibility if you have some knowledge of the programs, packages, and plans that are available. Although you should not recommend or endorse any specific program, book, diet, or organization, you can at least help your clients steer clear of dangerous fads, charlatans, and unscrupulous diet gurus.

How to Make Audio Recordings in Your Office

I previously recommended that you record the scripts (as you read them directly to the client) for sessions 5 through 8 of the WHY Program, and give the recordings to the client (see chapter 3). If you already have an audio-recording method for your sessions then the following paragraphs probably will not provide new information. However, if you've never recorded your sessions before, this information will get you started.

You can record your sessions on either audiotapes or CDs. Making a CD requires a few more steps and takes longer, but produces a longer-lasting recording. CDs also have the advantage that their content can be downloaded to various brands of MP3 players (and probably to whatever other audio technology gadgets may come along). Cassette tapes are rapidly becoming obsolete because they degrade with use or when exposed to heat, and the tape can break or unravel. To prevent the possibility that a client could accidentally push the "record" button on a cassette player and record over the tape, it is necessary to push in and break the tabs at the top of the cassette. Of course, ask if your client has a preference or equipment limitations.

The advantage of audiotapes is that they are easier to produce. All you need is a tape recorder, a blank tape (I recommend 45 minutes to a side) and a hand-held microphone plugged into the tape recorder. You can buy blank tapes (in clear plastic storage cases) in bulk from wholesale distributors for less than a dollar apiece. While recording, you could also operate a CD player in the background to play soothing music designed for hypnosis, relaxation, and meditation. You can purchase or download royalty-free music for this purpose from numerous web sites. If you keep the CD player close enough for the range of your microphone, you can tape the music as well as your voice.

To record an audio CD, you need the following:

- A computer with an internal CD burner disc drive. If you have an older computer that lacks or cannot accommodate an internal CD burner, you can purchase an external CD burner to plug into your computer via a USB connection.

- A digital audio recording device. This software capability is built in to some newer computers. With built-in recording capability, you can record directly into your computer by attaching a hand-held microphone to a microphone port on the computer. Another way to record is to use a hand-held digital voice recorder that has a self-contained microphone. I use an Olympus WS-100 that holds about five hours of recorded audio content. You can record into a digital voice recorder without attaching it to an electrical outlet or a computer, because the device runs on a battery. Whether you are using computer software or a hand-held recorder, you can have instant playback, with push-button controls for record, play, rewind, fast forward, and stop, just as on a tape recorder.

- Software on your computer for converting the audio file into a format that can be transferred to a CD. Nero and Roxio are popular brands of CD-burning software. If you know something about audio engineering, you can purchase software that allows you to edit and filter recordings (for example, to eliminate background noise).

- Blank CDs and jewel cases. Be sure to get CD-R (recordable) discs. You can buy blank CDs in bulk from any office supply store. Do not use CD-RWs (writable) because they are for storing data, not audio content. Unlike with cassette tapes, once you record audio to a CD-R, you cannot erase it, edit it, add more to the CD, or record over it. A CD-R holds about fifty to eighty minutes of audio content.

- Optional: An external audio content storage device. Audio files take up a lot of computer memory. If you want to store extra copies of your audio files, it's best to store them on an external memory device that holds a lot of memory. I am currently using a MicroGEM Quickie Drive with 4 GB of memory. It connects to my computer via a USB port.

There are two steps in recording an audio CD:

1. Record the session. If you are using a microphone connected to your computer, turn on the microphone and the computer and follow the software instructions. If you are using a digital voice recorder, turn it on and press "record." The recorder has a red light to indicate it is in "record" mode. Speak into the microphone or digital voice recorder to record your voice. Each time you press "stop" on the recorder then press "record" again, it creates a new track for the CD. When you have finished recording the session, press "stop."

2. Use audio conversion software on your computer to burn the audio recording onto a blank CD-R. Here are a few guidelines, but how you proceed really depends on the instructions for your particular software. First, if you have recorded your voice into a digital voice recorder, connect the recorder to your computer via the USB port. On your computer screen, you can find the audio file you have just created by accessing the USB drive, opening the drive, and then opening the folder with the file in it. Next, open up your audio software and follow the instructions in the software or the instruction manual for burning an audio file to a CD. Make sure the program is set to burn audio, not data or video, content. The software will allow you to select the audio file you wish to burn and the speed at which you want to

burn it. The program I use prompts me when to insert a blank CD into the CD burner drive. I click on the "burn" button, and the CD automatically pops out of the drive when the operation is complete.

The computer programmer I consulted for this section of the book advised a recording speed of 4x for voice quality. I've found that the transfer from audio file to CD takes about twelve minutes (but this will depend on your processor speed). As technology advances, these instructions may soon become incorrect or obsolete. The method you use to burn CDs will obviously depend on the type of computer you have and the software you are using. If you are not technology savvy, I recommend you engage the services of a computer technician who can show you the ropes. You can find one via personal recommendation, or go to the phone directory or the Internet and contact one of the "geek" companies that will send someone to your home or office to help you. Some computer stores provide in-store training or have employees who can give on-the-spot advice when you purchase your software or equipment.

By the way, when you are recording on audiotapes or CDs, it helps to have a permanent marker (the type that writes on plastic) to make a note of the contents right on the CD or cassette tape. Better still, you can pre-print adhesive labels with the content, your name, business address, phone number, and e-mail address to put on the finished product. At any office supply store you can purchase software and blank CD labels to type and print from your computer. For CDs, you will need a label applicator—just a plastic platform that allows you to press a label onto a CD without getting oily fingerprints on the recording side. Be sure to apply the label on the non-recording side of the CD.

Before you begin recording, make sure the client is seated or reclining comfortably. Having the client seated in a well-cushioned reclining chair works well. I offer my clients a neck pillow and a small blanket to place over their legs. I tell them they can remove their shoes or loosen their ties if they wish. You might want to promote a relaxing atmosphere by dimming the lights or burning a scented candle. Some practitioners I know use soothing aromatherapy scents while conducting hypnosis. Check that the client is agreeable and comfortable with your efforts at positive ambiance.

Setting Your Fee

Set your fee for the WHY Program based on your credentials, the ability of your selected clientele to pay the fee, and the general price standards of your profession in your locality. Keep in mind that the total fee generally includes the following:

- eight sessions of therapy (each at least an hour in length)

- four custom-made audiotapes or CDs
- client handouts
- any other take-home materials you might wish to provide

In addition to your usual operating expenses, your up-front costs for offering the program could include

- marketing materials and photocopying costs
- office forms and photocopying or printing costs
- audio-recording equipment and supplies

Here is a simple pricing strategy: Let's say you normally charge $100 for a one-hour session, and you plan to administer the program in eight one-hour sessions, for a total of $800. Let's say additionally that you charge $15 for each tape or CD, for a total of $60. Let's arbitrarily set the cost of printing off the *Client Workbook* at $5.00. The cost of the entire program now comes to $865.00.

You might also want to include some "extras" in your program. One example is a generic relaxation tape or CD—perhaps one you are reselling or have made and duplicated. A relaxation CD can serve as a stress management aid and a simple way to introduce your clients to the process of hypnosis. For my clients who are unfamiliar with hypnosis, I add a commercially available hypnotherapy relaxation CD as part of my program materials and add the cost to my fee. I buy these CDs in bulk at wholesale prices from the distributor. Other examples of "extras" are calorie counters, pulse-rate monitors, or recipe cards for low-calorie meals. Also consider articles, booklets, or reports you've written or obtained on topics relevant to weight control, goal setting, stress management, healthful lifestyles, positive thinking, motivation, or how to get the most from hypnotherapy.

You might also want to include a book or pamphlet with dietary guidelines. I include the book *Healthy Habits* in my offering. If you find a published book or commercial CD or DVD that you want to add to the WHY Program, you can usually buy it at a wholesale discount and sell it to your clients as part of the program at the retail price, folding the cost into your fee. You could also obtain free or low-cost public-information pamphlets on nutrition and exercise from government health organizations and pass those materials along to your clients at little or no cost as part of your "package."

If you are an approved care provider for a health maintenance organization, preferred provider organization, or health-care insurance organization and want to know how and whether you can bill your services to this organization, consult the representatives of the provider networks with which you are affiliated.

A Moment of Truth

How about you? Are you healthy and fit? Do you consistently eat healthful, wholesome foods; exercise; and maintain a healthy weight? If you can answer yes to these questions, congratulations! You are setting an excellent example for your clients. You need not read further in this chapter.

On the other hand, if you have excess weight, or you are not in great physical condition, it's time for a moment of truth—with yourself. As a practitioner, can you offer a credible weight reduction program if you are yourself contending with weight problems? Can you with integrity motivate any client to achieve a healthy weight limit if you have not done so yourself? You owe it to yourself and to your clients to set a healthy example. If you are not at a healthy weight, I recommend that you solve that problem before offering this program to your clients. Here are the steps to take:

- Consult your physician regarding your overall health, your target weight, a proper nutrition program, and the kinds of exercise appropriate for you. You might also consult a physical trainer or nutritionist or both.
- Start reading up on weight management and fitness.
- Implement a nutritional program and a safe, healthful physical exercise routine and stay with it.
- If you want group support in establishing a weight-management plan, join a reputable weight-management organization that offers sound advice on exercise and nutritional planning, under a program that makes sense to you.
- Find another NLP practitioner to conduct peer supervision with you. Ask this colleague to guide you through the WHY Program so that you can experience it for yourself. Complete all the sessions, listen to the tapes, read the take-home materials, practice self-hypnosis, and comply with the program guidelines.
- After the eight sessions, continue using all the tools. Stay with these changes until you have adopted new thought patterns and behaviors that will take you to your target weight and ensure you maintain it.
- If other issues arise around weight, food, and exercise, it is in your interest to return for additional individual sessions with your peer practitioner/ supervisor to access the resourceful states that will bring you optimal results.
- If additional medical issues arise, consult your physician and make the appropriate modifications in your food intake and exercise routine, in order to stay as healthy and active as possible.

Having achieved a healthy weight yourself, you'll have a valuable insight into the challenges your clients are facing. Drawing on the strategies that led to your successful results will be of tremendous benefit to your clients. I wish you motivation, determination, and much success!

Chapter 5

A Dozen Ways to Market the WHY Program

No therapeutic program in and of itself will bring clients to your practice. Now that you have invested in the WHY Program, naturally you are eager (I hope) to start using it with clients. This chapter contains twelve ways to market this program, so that more people find out about you, your practice, and how to reduce weight on the WHY Weight Reduction Program.

1. Offer a "free report" on hypnotherapy and weight reduction. You can tailor the sample report in appendix B to suit the unique aspects of your practice. You can circulate and distribute this report in the following ways:
   - Post it on your web site.
   - Offer it via e-mail or a URL in a newsletter about your practice that you send to clients and colleagues.
   - Staple your business card to a paper copy of the report and offer it to your current clients when they come in for sessions. Just say, "This article tells you about a new service I'm offering—hypnotherapy for weight reduction. If you know of anyone who could use this service, please pass it along to him or her."
   - Place several copies of the report in your waiting room for clients to read and take home.
   - Mail the report to physicians in your area with a cover letter describing your credentials and the services you offer. Enclose your business card.

2. Post your WHY Program brochure (see appendix D for a sample) on community bulletin boards (with management permission) in local spas, health clubs, and weight reduction centers.

3. Offer a free thirty-minute talk to local groups concerned with good health. You could give this talk to women's groups, community education organizations, local civic groups, and health clubs. Hand out your business card and WHY Program brochure to attendees. In terms of a general outline, your talk could cover the following points:
   - who you are: your credentials, the scope of your practice, and your specialized training in hypnotherapy and NLP
   - an explanation of hypnotherapy and NLP
   - how hypnotherapy and NLP can be an important part of a healthful weight reduction program

- • an overview of the WHY Program
- • some success stories (maintaining confidentiality, of course).

4. Offer to speak to community college and university classes of students in the fields of counseling, psychology, social work, and nursing. Talk about the practice of NLP and hypnotherapy and related applications, including weight reduction. These students may be future referral sources for you or may come to you for supervision. Hand out your business card and brochures, and give the students an opportunity to sign up for your electronic newsletter if you have one.

5. Contact the staff at your local public-access television station or a local radio station and ask if they welcome guest speakers on "community interest" or "health-oriented" programs. If there is a program on which you might want to appear, ask for the program producer's contact information. Approach the producer about being a guest on the program to talk about hypnotherapy, NLP, and health management/weight reduction. Ask about the format of the show, and tailor your talk to it. Prepare well for the show in order to appear at your best. Afterwards, send thank-you notes to the staff, the producer, and the host.

6. Get a booth or table at a local health fair or community fitness day event. Hand out the free report on hypnotherapy and weight reduction. Have plenty of business cards and brochures to give away. People will often drop by your table and talk with you if you have a small gift to offer—perhaps a fifteen-minute relaxation tape or a drawing for a prize (a book or videotape on self-improvement), or a rate-yourself quiz on hypnotizability or some other trait. When people stop at your table, engage them and tell them about your practice. If you cannot afford the cost of a table, share the table and the cost with a colleague in a related field.

7. Contact local weight-control clinics and doctors' offices in your area. I recommend you meet mostly with those physicians and medical personnel who have occasion to treat overweight clients: bariatricians, orthopedists, physical therapists, chiropractors, gynecologists, nutritionists, and endocrinologists, for example. Ask to meet with the management or staff to tell them about your practice and the WHY Program, and to ask for their referrals.

By the way, when you receive referrals from health practitioners, acknowledge these referrals with thank-you cards and gifts. For example, a nearby obstetrics and gynecology practice regularly refers clients to me for weight reduction and stress management. In return, I send thank-you cards and seasonal gift baskets to the office staff. Because the clinic is a health practice,

I refrain from sending baskets containing sweets and alcohol. Instead, I send baskets of fruits, low-calorie cheeses, and nuts.

8. Place your ad in the telephone directory under the heading for "weight control" or "weight reduction" or "weight loss." Offer a "free phone consultation," and when prospects call, tell them about the WHY Program. Offer to mail a brochure or a free report.

9. On your phone or voice-mail greeting, include more than your name and "leave a message." Use your recording to advertise! Here is an example:

    > Hello, you've reached Motivational Strategies, offering solution-oriented counseling featuring hypnotherapy and NLP. Ask about special programs for weight control, smoking cessation, and pain management. Please leave your name and number and a short message, so I can return your call. Thank you for calling.

10. As you develop a client base, collect testimonials from satisfied clients who have completed the WHY Program. Include these in your marketing materials and on your web site.

11. Team up with a nutritionist, personal trainer, or other fitness expert. Offer via the Internet a free forty-five- to sixty-minute class on fitness, weight control, stress management, and exercise. Schedule the times and dates for the class and advertise it well in advance, via e-mail, electronic newsletters, web site announcements, and word of mouth. Tell people how to dial up the class. During the class, discuss the efficacy of hypnotherapy for weight reduction and talk about the WHY Program.

12. After a client completes the WHY Program and has had a satisfying experience, send a follow-up letter with a WHY Program brochure enclosed. (Find a sample follow-up letter in appendix E.) The purpose of this letter is
    *   to wish the client continued success in weight reduction
    *   to offer additional services
    *   to ask the client to refer friends who might benefit from the WHY Program

There you have it: one dozen ways to market the WHY Program. Although these methods are all relatively inexpensive, they do require time and planning. As a practitioner in private practice or in a group practice, chances are you are already doing some similar marketing activities. Therefore, these suggestions may dovetail with your current marketing schedule. Use the methods that work best for you, considering your marketing budget, your available time, your referral network, and your locale.

A few final words about marketing are in order: Many therapists are reluctant to market their practices because they don't want to be a salesperson. They consider their work a calling rather than just "a job." They don't want to be "pushy" or self-promoting, because those characteristics are not consistent with the image we all hope to project of a compassionate, sincere, caring, helping professional. So how do we get around this dilemma to let potential clients know that we exist and that we have something to offer?

Lynn Grodski, social worker, business coach, and author of the book *Building Your Ideal Private Practice* (2000), advises therapists to use "pull" marketing instead of "push" marketing. "Push" marketing promotes a product that people may or may not need, whereas "pull" marketing offers solutions to a select group of prospects who have a specific problem. "Push" marketing uses a shotgun approach, advertising impersonally to the general public. "Pull" marketing is sensitive, respectful, and professional, ensuring a safe, ethical, and confidential approach. Instead of mass mailings or an advertising campaign, you market your practice via relationship skills. Build a solid referral network based on personal contacts through former and existing clients and people in your e-mail address book, people who have inquired about your work, colleagues, and people whom you have met face-to-face. Perfect your social and conversational skills and believe in what you do passionately and enthusiastically. Ask for referrals and thank those who send you referrals with a personal note. Let your confidence and enthusiasm show whenever and wherever you talk about your work—and the clients will come.

Part II

Conducting the Eight Sessions of the WHY Program

Chapter 6

Session 1: Intake Interview and Introduction to the WHY Program

Purpose

In the initial session you familiarize your client with the WHY Program. This is often your first opportunity to establish rapport with clients and talk to them face-to-face about their weight reduction goals and how the program will help them. In this session you want to make sure the client has a complete understanding of the program and its requirements, as well as healthy, reasonable expectations about what weight reduction results are possible and what hypnotherapy can accomplish. Additionally, you want to assess your client's commitment to weight reduction and to attending all eight sessions. This is also your opportunity to tell your client about your approach to hypnosis and NLP and to respond to the client's questions and concerns.

Procedures

Clinical Interview

1. Have the client read, complete, and sign any paperwork you require, such as your client information/identification forms, privacy statement, payment agreement, and informed consent agreement.

2. Conduct and document your clinical interview. I recommend that you inquire about the following:
    *   the client's background and current life circumstances
    *   the client's overall emotional health, life stresses, and coping skills
    *   the client's sleep patterns
    *   the client's problems with food and weight management and the changes he or she wants to make
    *   the client's weight reduction goals and expectations about your work
    *   whether the client has consulted a physician concerning an appropriate target weight, an appropriate nutrition plan, and appropriate kinds of exercise. Make sure the client is participating in a medically supervised or physician-approved dietary or nutrition plan throughout the duration of the WHY Program

- any medical problems or issues that might call for modifications to the scripted suggestions in this book (dietary restrictions or exercise restrictions, for example)
- any medical or mental-health issues that could contraindicate participation in the WHY Program (see chapter 3)
- previous experience with NLP, hypnotherapy, or psychotherapy. If the client has previous experience, ascertain what was and was not helpful.
- other concerns that might help you in understanding and working effectively with this client
- the client's prior experience with weight reduction methods: What worked and what did not?
- any current problems with substance abuse (illegal drugs, prescription drugs, inhalants, or alcohol). This factor is a serious contraindication that could undermine the client's success in weight reduction.
- the client's relationship with significant others who may or may not be supportive of the client's weight reduction goals.

Program Overview

1. Give the client an overview of the WHY Program. Explain its purpose and summarize each of the eight sessions. Make sure the client understands the requirement and rationale for (a) advance payment with no refund; (b) attending all eight sessions; and (c) reducing at least four pounds (two kilos) after each of sessions 4, 5, 6, and 7, for a total of at least sixteen pounds (or eight kilos) by session 8.

2. Explain that the hypnotherapy portions of sessions 5 through 8 will be audio-recorded. The client receives these recordings and is encouraged to reinforce his or her progress through listening to each session as many times as desired. Go over the cautions and caveats regarding the use of these audio recordings (see appendix C: "Sample Informed Consent Agreement").

3. Give the client any brochures you have developed that might be helpful in explaining the WHY Program or information about you and your practice that you want your clients to know. Appendix D contains a sample brochure on the WHY Program that you can use as a model for creating your own brochure.

4. Briefly explain the processes of hypnotherapy and NLP and answer any questions or concerns the client may have about your approach. Appendixes G and H contain two articles, "Introduction to Clinical Hypnosis and Hypnotherapy" and "What Is Neuro-Linguistic Programming?" which you may photocopy and give to your client as take-home materials.

Agree on Outcomes

Ensure that you and your client are in agreement as to well-formed behavioral outcomes. The outcomes could specify changes the client will make in eating, portion control, food selection, food preparation, and exercise in order to achieve a reduction of at least sixteen pounds (eight kilos) by session 8. To be safe, the client should generally slim down by no more than two pounds a week. Make sure the client's goals are realistic and put them in writing so that you and the client can review them in the future.

Optional: Obtain Permission to Share the Client's Information

Ask whether your client is working with other health-care practitioners and wishes you to share with them relevant information about his or her progress in the WHY Program. These other health practitioners could include the client's physician, nutritionist, holistic medicine practitioner, clinical nurse practitioner, massage therapist, chiropractor, allergist, psychiatrist, couples counselor, pastoral counselor, or other specialist. If the client wants you to share information with another practitioner, have the client sign your release or exchange of information form, indicating the name, address, and phone number of the practitioner with whom you will share the information. I recommend that you not share such information via e-mail, unless you can guarantee a secure e-mail connection that protects the client's privacy.

Sharing information with other health-care practitioners serves many purposes:

- The practitioner could give you additional insights and background information about your client and how best to work with him or her.
- The practitioner could agree to support the client in his or her weight reduction goals and encourage the client to participate fully in the WHY Program.
- You can answer the practitioner's questions about the WHY Program, and establish your credentials and credibility.
- You become a member of the client's health-care team.

Optional: Conduct Tests of Hypnotizability

Some practitioners routinely conduct tests of hypnotizability and others do not. I do if the client questions whether he or she can be hypnotized, or if the client tells me of previous problems with being hypnotized. If you wish to conduct tests of hypnotizability and you don't have a method that you already use, here are some recommendations:

With the client's permission, conduct one or two tests or indicators of suggestibility or hypnotizability to (a) reassure the client he or she can be hypnotized and (b) ascertain how the client follows your instructions. You can select from the many tests that are well documented in hypnotherapy books and manuals. Such tests include arm levitation; the finger magnets test; the Speigel (1972) eye-roll test; or the light hand, heavy hand test. Author and hypnotherapist Tad James (James, Flores, and Schober 2000) refers to the last test as the "dictionary and balloon test." Tests such as these go by various names depending on the text you read. Two good sources are James, Flores, and Schober (2000) and Allen (2004). You may want to administer a paper-and-pencil test such as the Stanford Hypnosis Susceptibility Scale (Weitzenhoffer and Hilgard 1963) or the Hypnotic Induction Profile (Stern, Speigel, and Nee 1979), if you find such measures useful.

The client's response to these tests will give you some idea about his or her degree of comfort and cooperation in working with you so that you can modify your approach accordingly. For example, does the client tend to match or mismatch instructions? You might also conduct a brief hypnotic induction and reorientation, if time permits, to familiarize the client with the hypnotic process.

If your client exhibits little hypnotizability, you could conduct an extra session focused on enhancing his or her hypnotizability. Experiment with various induction methods to discover which types seem to work best for the client. Perhaps an even better option is to give the client a generic hypnotic relaxation audiotape or CD with which to practice at home, to improve hypnotizability. Such audiotapes or CDs can be purchased commercially, or you can make your own and duplicate it. This tape or CD should be instructive in nature, teaching the client how to relax deeply, become familiar with trance, accept suggestions for deepening, and improve susceptibility to hypnosis. By the way, for the hypnotic procedures you use in these eight sessions, you might refer to appendix F, "Eighteen Ways to Induce and Deepen Hypnotic Trance."

Obtain the Client's Commitment

1. Obtain the client's commitment to the WHY Program and build his or her response potential. A sample dialogue might go like this:

    You've told me you want to reduce your weight, and you are willing to invest money and time in doing so. I know you want to succeed.

    As you make behavioral changes, you will probably begin to eat less of the foods that have been problematic for you. You'll also want to start an exercise plan, if you haven't done so already.

I want to work only with people I believe are really committed to this endeavor. If you know of any circumstances that would keep you from full participation in this program, I want you to discuss them with me, so that we can find solutions now. If you have any hesitations or reservations about our work together, let me know now, so that we can work those out together.

This program does not work for everyone, and one of the main reasons why people fail is that they are not fully committed. They give the assignments a halfhearted attempt or don't follow a food plan or don't listen to the recordings or don't find time to exercise, and they expect this program to be just another failure that proves they can't lose weight. Now if any of these factors describes your situation, please tell me now, so that we can discuss whether this is the right move for you at this time.

A full commitment to your outcome would entail the following:

- Attend all eight sessions.

- Work with a safe, healthy nutrition plan.

- Start and continue a safe, healthful exercise routine.

- Be honest about reducing your weight by four pounds (or two kilos) after each of sessions 4, 5, 6, and 7.

- Listen to the audio recordings.

- Read the materials and complete each take-home assignment prior to returning for the following session.

Are you willing to do these things?

2. If the client isn't certain of his or her commitment at this point, ask, "Can you think of anything that might prevent you from participating in this program? Can you think of anything that might prevent you from getting the results you want?"

   These questions will usually surface any concerns, worries, fears, or limitations that might undermine successful outcomes. Address these obstacles thoroughly and help the client decide whether they can be surmounted and, if so, help the client develop a workable plan. If not, perhaps it would best for the client to withdraw from the program for now.

3. When you obtain the client's commitment, reinforce it in this way. Ask, "How do you know when you are committed to some endeavor or some plan? How does it feel when you know you are ready to give your all?" Encourage the client to apply the same level of commitment and readiness to the WHY Program. If the client doesn't feel that full level of commitment, again, help the client identify how the program could meet his or her criteria and develop a workable plan.

Elicit an Outcome Chain

An outcome chain (Andreas and Andreas 1994) is a hierarchy of increasingly valued outcome states associated with doing, having, and being. Eliciting an outcome chain helps your client link higher-level values to program outcomes and thus enrich his or her commitment to it. Begin the process by asking about the client's primary motivating value in achieving and maintaining a healthy weight. Most people will say they want to be healthy, because this is the socially acceptable answer. It sounds right, but if it were compelling, that person wouldn't be sitting in your office, taking up more than enough space on the chair. There are two ways to make values compelling. One is to move a value from an abstraction into a see-hear-feel representation. Another way is to link a value to values higher up in the individual's hierarchy. Practitioners elicit values because the mind generally stores them at the subconscious level. If you tell the average person, "List your values and put them in order of priority," most would be stumped.

To elicit an outcome chain, follow these steps:

1. Ask about the client's primary value attached to eating properly, exercising, and reducing weight: "What is so vital and important about reducing your weight that you are willing to eat or exercise properly and consistently for as long as it takes to get the results you want?"

2. Take the client's answer and ask the client to describe it as a see-hear-feel representation. What does it look like, sound like, and feel like to be healthy? Now describe it back to the client and ask the client to associate to the experience you describe.

3. Ask the client, "Now that you can imagine this experience, if you could have this experience of health, fully and completely, in this way, then what would be so valuable about it that it would be even more meaningful and significant than health itself?"

4. Continue to elicit the client's additional values in the same way, until the client describes a highly valued core state. The core state is ineffable and often spiritual. Examples are "oneness" or "peace" or "completeness" or "fulfillment." Sometimes when people reach the core state in the outcome chain, they say they can't think of anything beyond that state, or they may loop back to a previous state in an effort to make sense of the request for yet another higher-order value.

5. Invite the client to associate to the core state. Establish an anchor for the core state. Reverse the outcome chain, applying the anchor, bringing it to bear as a Meta-State on the previous outcomes in the chain.

6. Finally, bring the core state to bear on full participation in all aspects of the WHY Program. Now have the client associate to a representation of feeling healthy and attractive at the target weight and describe the state again in see-hear-feel terms, this time applying the anchor from the core state in the outcome chain.

NLP trainers Connirae and Tamara Andreas have described how to elicit an outcome chain in detail in their book *Core Transformation* (1994). Here is a short sample dialogue to illustrate how eliciting an "outcome chain" might progress.

Practitioner: What is it about reducing your weight that is so valuable to you?

Client: I'd be healthier. (Preliminary outcome)

Practitioner: Describe to me what being healthy is all about for you. Give me some specific examples.

Client: Having energy to take a walk or climb a flight of stairs. Not getting winded and out of breath. Moving around more easily—more coordination. Not looking so flabby. Looking and feeling more attractive. Hearing someone tell me I'm looking healthier—maybe that I look younger.

Practitioner: Step into that way of feeling and being. Full of energy and vitality, moving easily and freely, taking a walk and swinging your arms with a bounce in your step, going up a staircase and feeling okay—feeling fit—moving easily. Really feel it. Feel good when you look at yourself in the mirror and see less flab and more lean. You might be saying to yourself, "Wow! I look good, and I feel light and energetic." Imagine a loved one or friend telling you that you look healthier and younger. How do you feel with these experiences? Now that you know what feeling healthy is like, and if you could have this experience of health, fully and completely, in this way, then what would be so valuable about it that would make it even more meaningful and significant than health itself?

Client: Self-esteem—feeling good about myself, feeling confident and attractive. (Preliminary outcome)

Practitioner: Okay, step into that situation of feeling confident and attractive. You get up in the morning feeling good about yourself—liking yourself—being okay with who you are—your smarts, talents, skills, and capabilities. Even say, "Hey! I like myself. I'm feeling good about just being me." Maybe you have a lightness in your heart, a smile on your face, a song in your head, and a bounce in your step. Life feels easier! Imagine it now. If you could have all that, fully and completely, what is it about having self-esteem that is even more valuable than self-esteem itself?

Client: Feeling complete—at one with myself—peaceful. (Core state)

Practitioner: Think of times and places in your life where you have felt moments of true peace. Where you've felt totally complete—at one with yourself and the universe. Remember how that peace feels now. Close your eyes and move into that feeling—complete, at one with yourself, peaceful. Hear the words in your mind—peaceful, calm, tranquil, and serene. Make those feelings full and profound. Have them totally. See, hear, and feel the meaning of "complete" peacefulness—the sense of oneness with self.

57

Bring that feeling of completeness, oneness, and peace into the concept of enhanced self-esteem ... a more complete self-esteem, a more peaceful self-esteem ... fuller, more satisfying than before ... loving, liking and taking care of yourself, so very okay with who you are that it enhances all you do.

And bring that same deeper, fuller completeness, oneness, and peace into the idea of health. See the glow of health around you. Feel the glow, the energy, the vitality. Moving easily and freely and feeling complete, at one, and full of peace at every level of mind and body. Walking, bending, stretching, moving more into feeling complete, at one with yourself, peaceful in a healthy, fit body.

Your commitment and motivation are enhanced as you find that, more than ever, you enjoy healthy eating patterns, healthful foods, and healthful activity, and you are sticking with the program, staying with your plan, getting to your target weight. How much more motivated do you feel now?

Wrap-up

Collect your fee, give the client a receipt, and schedule the next session. You are free to make copies of appendix G: "Introduction to Clinical Hypnosis and Hypnotherapy" and appendix H: "What Is Neuro-Linguistic Programming?" and give these to the client, if you wish.

Client assignment for session 1: Give the client the take-home assignment for session 1: "Get the Results You Want: Well-Formed Outcomes for Weight Control," on the *Client Workbook* CD.

Practitioner Checklist and Notes

Session 1: Intake Interview and Introduction to the WHY Program

Copy, complete, and put in the client's file.

Checklist	Notes
Client's name: _____ Date of session: _____ ❑ Have the client sign any paperwork, such as an identification form and informed consent agreement. ❑ Conduct a clinical interview. ❑ Give an overview of the WHY Program. ❑ Give any brochures on your practice. ❑ List the client's well-formed outcomes. ❑ Optional: Obtain the client's signature on a release/exchange of information form. ❑ Optional: Conduct tests of hypnotizability. ❑ Obtain the client's commitment. ❑ Explain clinical hypnosis and NLP. Optional take-home materials: appendixes G: "Introduction to Clinical Hypnosis and Hypnotherapy" and H: "What Is Neuro-Linguistic Programming?" ❑ Give *Client Workbook* assignment for session 1: "Get the Results You Want: Well-Formed Outcomes for Weight Control." ❑ Collect the fee for the entire program.	

Chapter 7

Session 2: Reframing Compulsive Eating

Purpose

Reframing is the process of developing (or helping the client develop) new meanings and understandings about an unwanted behavior. In this session you will use the Six-Step Reframe (sometimes called a content reframe) to help the client identify at least one internal motivation that prompts overeating or unnecessary eating (that is, eating when one is not really hungry).

The Six-Step Reframe was developed by Richard Bandler and John Grinder (1982). It is based on the concepts associated with ego state therapy (Emmerson 2003) in which the human personality is characterized as a collection of sub-personalities, or "parts," called ego states, each with its own function or purpose. When people feel congruent, all their ego states are working together in an integrated fashion. When people feel incongruent, as when they persist in an unwanted habit, it is because some ego state, or part of self, is behaving in a way that is out of harmony with the rest of the ego states that comprise the "sense of self."

According to one of the premises of NLP, all parts within an individual's personality serve a positive intention—usually satisfying basic human physical and emotional needs, or upholding values and beliefs. In theory, then, we could say that "parts" influence actions and behaviors intended to fulfill positive intentions, even when the intentions are known only at a subconscious level.

Parts sometimes prompt unwanted or hurtful or self-harming behaviors in attempts to satisfy positive intentions. Paradoxically, these hurtful behaviors sometimes cause the very problems they are intended to prevent. Often, as in the case of overeating, the positive intention may be to provide comfort or relieve stress. Even though wolfing down a bag of chocolate chip cookies can bring a momentary sense of well-being or pleasure, the resulting regret and disgust can be very uncomfortable, and the resulting weight gain can be a source of additional discomfort and stress.

The Six-Step Reframe helps you and the client contact the client's "part of self" responsible for overeating, identify the positive intention behind overeating or binging, and persuade that part to choose alternatives to overeating. I like to tell my clients that this is a method that takes all the energy attached to overeating and channels that energy in a new, healthier direction.

Procedure

Begin by following up on the previous session. Obtain feedback and respond to any questions or concerns the client may have. Then give an overview of session 2 and conduct the Six-Step Reframe, as described below.

Six-Step Reframe

Explain that the purpose of this session is to help the client identify the underlying and often unconscious dynamics of overeating or binging. This method enhances the client's ability to control runaway eating patterns. It helps the client examine an unwanted behavior or habit from a new perspective and, metaphorically, to communicate with a part of self that is causing the problem behavior. Here are the steps. Note: For each step, ask the client to close the eyes, complete the step, and then open the eyes. Clients who do not wish to close their eyes can simply stare at a blank surface such as a wall, a door, or the ceiling. A sample script is provided.

1. *Identify the Part*

    a. Introduce the "parts" frame:

    > Sometimes when people repeatedly do things they regret, or wish they didn't do, but they can't seem to stop themselves, we could say that a "part of self" is prompting the unwanted behavior. I want to teach you a method for contacting the part of your self that has led you to overeat, identify the part's positive intention for you, and ask that part to find alternative ways to satisfy the intention, so that you can channel that energy in more positive directions.

    b. Teach the client how to establish inner contact with the part.

    > In a moment I'm going to ask you to relax, close your eyes, and mentally invite that "part" into your conscious awareness. There's no right or wrong way to do this. It is an intuitive process, so just be open and receptive to your inner experience. The part will make itself known to you in one of many ways. Perhaps it will be an image in your mind, such as a symbol, an object, or a memory. Or it might be something you feel on a physical level—a sensation. It might be some inner dialogue—something you say to yourself. Whatever you experience will be just fine. Now make yourself comfortable, take a deep breath, relax, close your eyes, and go ahead. When you have some indication from that part, open your eyes and we'll talk about it.

c. Wait quietly for the client to complete this step. When the client opens his or her eyes, ask about the inner experience. How did the client inwardly represent the part? When the client has identified the part, suggest that the client thank the part for its cooperation: "Inwardly thank that part for making itself known to you in this way."

Troubleshooting tips: On rare occasions I've had a client who reports having no internal experience and no indication of a part. In this case, I ask the client to imagine what the part might look like. Then I ask the client to visualize the part in the palm of his or her hand, or sitting in an empty chair across the room. This variation seems to help clients who may have a problem reporting on internal representations.

2. *Calibrate Yes and No from the Part*

   a. Help the client establish communication with the part:

   > Close your eyes again and ask the part if it is willing to communicate with you. When you receive an answer—yes or no—from the part, open your eyes and tell me the answer you received.

   b. Wait quietly while the client completes this step. When the client opens his or her eyes, ask, "What occurred that indicated a yes or no answer to you?" My experience has been that some clients think this step is an invitation to begin analyzing themselves or explaining the problem. I have found it important to remind the client that the desired response from the part is simply yes or no.

   c. If the client tells you the answer is yes, then say:

   > Close your eyes again and reconnect with that part. Thank the part for saying yes, for indicating that it is willing to communicate with you. Now ask that part to demonstrate a response that indicates no, so that it is able to indicate both yes and no.

   d. Wait for the client to complete this step, then go on to step 3.

Troubleshooting tips: If the client's initial response is no, explore ecological concerns and the client's understanding of the procedure. When the client conveys a no response, I have found it's usually because the client has taken an adversarial attitude toward the part. Some clients have told me they want to "get rid of" the part or "get even" with it. In that case, explain that the process is a "part-friendly" one in which the client has an opportunity to appreciate what the part is trying to do and negotiate with it.

After exploring ecological concerns and explaining the process more thoroughly, tell the client, "Close your eyes and ask if the part is now willing to communicate with you." Again, wait for the client to complete this step and open his or her eyes. Usually, the answer this time will be yes. If so, tell the client to appreciate the part for cooperating. If the response remains no, consider abandoning this method and using an alternative method in your NLP or hypnosis repertoire (see chapter 16 for additional NLP patterns for overeating).

3. *Identify the Positive Intention*

   a. Ask the client to reconnect with the part and find out the positive intention behind overeating:

      Close your eyes again and reconnect with the part. Ask the part to tell you the positive intention behind overeating. In other words, what does the part want to do for you by causing you to overeat? Just relax now and let the answer come to you. Open your eyes when you have the answer.

   b. Wait quietly for the client to complete this step. When the client opens his or her eyes, ask what he or she represented as the positive intention. Help the client appreciate the positive intention.

   Troubleshooting tips: Sometimes the client's response will indicate a very clear, logical intention. At other times the client's response is vague and seemingly irrelevant. In the latter case, it is up to you to help the client flesh out the meaning of the response and figure out the positive intention. Somehow there usually is a connection.

   Sometimes the client gives a response that suggests a negative intention instead of a positive one. Your reply should be, "And what would *that* do for you?" Keep asking until you get a positive intention. For example, a client once told me the intention of overeating was "to make me die." When I asked "What would *dying* do for you?" her reply was, "So I could go to heaven and be happy." I then inquired, "Are there other ways for you to go to heaven without having to overeat? Are there other ways to be happy now, without having to wait until you die?"

4. *Help the Client Find Alternatives to Satisfy the Positive Intention*

   a. Explain to the client that parts often get stuck in a rut, using ineffective or harmful methods to satisfy a positive intention and not knowing what else to do. It helps to give such parts a wider repertoire, or more flexibility—sort of an upgrade in the part's job description. Tell the client that you are going to give that part instructions so that it can access the client's inner resources—such as creativity, intuition, and inner wisdom—and can consider alternatives to overeating.

Now close your eyes again and as you relax, reconnect with that part. It may seem the same, or it may seem different somehow. We want this part to understand that overeating does not really solve the problem or satisfy the positive intention, and overeating in this way is actually harmful and unhealthy. So now this part has an opportunity to do its job more effectively, with more flexibility.

Tell this part you are giving it full access to your inner resources, such as your creativity, your intuition, and your inner wisdom, so that it can begin to learn more than ever before. The part can access these inner resources right now, even as I am speaking to you. As this part is learning and improving, it can begin to create a list or a survey of additional ways to accomplish that positive intention—healthy, convenient ways to do it ... numerous options and alternatives to overeating, so that overeating is no longer the only choice ... and that energy gets channeled into more positive pursuits.

As that part of yourself begins to register all these options and alternatives, it can select three of those options and bring them into your conscious awareness for your review and approval. So when those three selections ... those alternatives ... are available to you, open your eyes.

b. Wait quietly while the client completes this step. When the client's eyes are open, ask about the three selections. Evaluate with the client whether these selections are realistic and suitable for satisfying the positive intention. At least one of these choices should be easy and convenient to do—offering the same ease and convenience as food. Encourage the client to appreciate the creativity that brought these selections forth and to notice how well the part is cooperating.

Troubleshooting tips: Some clients do not think of three alternatives. They might, instead, think of only one or two. Some clients think of four or five alternatives. Whatever number of alternatives the client produces, accept them and tell the client he or she is doing good work.

If the client can't think of any alternatives, brainstorm together until you jointly produce three suitable alternatives to overeating that will satisfy the positive intention.

Remember this process does not rule out the choice to overeat. Do not say anything to the effect that overeating is no longer an option. The purpose of this reframe is to expand choices, not eliminate them. A client could still on occasion choose to overeat, but will be aware of other choices. A client of mine used this process to decide that she would eat sweets only one night a week, and the rest of the week, she would engage in other, healthier activities for self-soothing.

Occasionally, I've had clients who misunderstand this step as an instruction to find ways to thwart the behavior of overeating, instead of to satisfy the positive intention in a different way. For example: "I could tell my husband to stop bringing home potato chips" instead of, "I could find other ways to cope with stress, such as listening to my favorite music." Be sure your client clearly understands this step and completes it.

5. *Enter into a Contract with the Part*

    a. Instruct the client to make a contract or agreement with the part to choose one of the healthier alternatives whenever there is a need to fill the positive intention that led to overeating:

        Close your eyes and relax again and thank that part for selecting those alternatives. Know you have additional ways to take care of yourself and meet your needs. I ask you now to enter into a contract with that part, such that from now on, whenever you need to satisfy that intention (e.g., cope with stress, comfort yourself, etc.), that part will automatically choose one of these healthier alternatives. In fact, should that part require even more flexibility, it can continue to access your creativity, your intuition, and your inner wisdom to arrive at additional healthy, positive choices that will serve your needs and desires.

        When that part is in agreement with this contract, nod your head. On the other hand, if that part has any reservations or concerns, open your eyes and let's talk about them.

    b. Wait quietly until the client is ready. If the client nods, go on to step 6. If the client expresses reservations or concerns, explore these. Offer reassurances and help the client think of modifications, exceptions, or alternatives, as needed, to address any ecological issues. When the client is satisfied that all concerns have been addressed, go on to step 6.

6. *Future Rehearsal*

    a. Have the client mentally review the new alternatives to overeating:

        Close your eyes again and thank that part for entering into the contract with you. See images in which you are choosing suitable, healthy ways to take care of yourself. Step into those images one by one and enjoy the new behaviors.

    b. Guide the client through possible future scenarios in which he or she is choosing one or more of the alternatives selected in step 4, in order to satisfy the positive intention. Here is a sample of what you might say:

        Let's say you've come home from a challenging day at the office, and you want to take some time to relax and pamper yourself (the positive intention). You sit down in the easy chair in the den, and you begin to listen to your favorite music (one of the alternatives to overeating). As you close your eyes and relax, a sense of contentment comes over you, and all the cares and frustrations of the day seem to melt away and you feel so much more at ease. You are quite pleased and satisfied that you have found this method of pampering yourself.

Wrap-up

1. Reorient the client to wakeful alertness.

2. Conclude your session with the client and schedule session 3.

Client assignment for session 2: Give the client the take-home assignment for session 2: "Trim-Slim Thinking versus Fat Thinking" on the *Client Workbook* CD.

Practitioner Checklist and Notes

Session 2: Reframing Compulsive Eating

Copy, complete, and put in the client's file.

Checklist	Notes
Client's name: _____ Date of session: _____ ❏ Follow up on any questions or concerns from the previous session. ❏ Ask the client about any questions on the previous session's take-home assignment: "Get the Results You Want: Well-Formed Outcomes for Weight Control" from the *Client Workbook* CD. ❏ Explain and conduct the Six-Step Reframe, noting the positive intention(s) that overeating fills and the alternatives to overeating. ❏ Give the client the take-home assignment for session 2: "Trim-Slim Thinking versus Fat Thinking."	

Chapter 8

Session 3: Training in Self-Hypnosis

Purpose

The purpose of the third session is to teach the client self-hypnosis, so that he or she feels empowered to initiate and manage change, develop solution-oriented thinking patterns, visualize success, and replace unwanted behaviors with more effective alternatives. Learning self-hypnosis reassures the client that trance is a naturally occurring state of mind and that hypnosis is not magical or mystical. It reveals that the client has the capacity to create change and makes him or her an ally with you in the therapeutic process.

Procedure

1. Before the session, familiarize yourself with the assignment for session 3 in the *Client Workbook*: "Learning Self-Hypnosis—The Seven-Step Self-Hypnosis Process." You'll find a sample self-hypnosis template at the end of this chapter, which you can photocopy and use as a worksheet for this session.

2. Before you begin teaching self-hypnosis, ask the client about progress or problems since the last session. Discuss what's working and what isn't, commending progress and new understandings and addressing any concerns.

3. Explain that the reason for learning self-hypnosis is so that the client can become an active participant in the change process, learning more about how hypnosis works and how to use hypnosis to focus positive thoughts on specific outcomes. Here is an example of what you might say:

    The purpose of learning self-hypnosis is so that you can manage your own thoughts more effectively and guide your own progress. Self-hypnosis helps you concentrate on large and small outcomes by talking to yourself about them in positive ways, and by visualizing how you want to think, feel, and act to create specific results. It is a way of tuning in to your own potential so that you come to believe in your ability to steer your own course and rely on your inner resources to be there for you.

Think about this: If you have been doing a lot of negative self-talk about food and weight and that sort of thing, it has probably made you feel depressed or frustrated—and it only reinforced the problem. You could say you were hypnotizing yourself in this very nonproductive way for a long time. Now you can turn it around and get your thoughts and energies going in a positive direction.

You can be very flexible with self-hypnosis. You can do it in five minutes a day—say when you first wake up in the morning. Or you could use it when you want a boost of motivation and confidence, say, for example, before going to a party, so that you can make sure you choose the veggies at the buffet.

The take-home assignment for this session will even give you a short script so that you can audio-record your own hypnosis scripts and listen to them at home.

Today, I'm going to teach you an easy seven-step process for designing your own self-hypnosis sessions. With practice, you can vary the way you do it. There is no wrong or right way to do self-hypnosis. The worksheet is an example of just one method. You can eventually add your own variations that work for you. The more you learn about self-hypnosis, the more you tap into the power of your inner resources. After you learn the seven steps, then for the remainder of the session I'll teach you some easy methods for going into trance and coming out of trance again, all by yourself.

The Seven-Step Self-Hypnosis Process

If you have a method you prefer for teaching your clients self-hypnosis, use your method instead of mine. If you want to employ my method, or some variation thereof, here are the seven steps of the self-hypnosis process as I teach it to my clients. Each step is addressed to the client, so "you" throughout the following instructions refers to the client. The template I use is shown in assignment 3 of the *Client Workbook*. At the end of this chapter is an identical template that you can photocopy to use as a worksheet.

1. Identify the problem or concern you want to address and plan it on your template (steps 1 and 3–6). You can copy the template to create as many as you wish.

2. Induce trance. There are many ways to get into a state of focused concentration. Use one that works for you.

3. Now focus on what you will do as your solution—imagine how you will think, feel, and act.

4. Visualize yourself carrying out the new behavior. This is your mental rehearsal.

5. State positive affirmations that you can easily repeat to yourself to remind yourself about the changes you are creating.

6. Now make your own posthypnotic suggestion with this easy formula: "From now on when I encounter X, I am doing Y."

7. Reorient yourself: open your eyes if they were closed, stretch, and take a deep breath. Done!

Make sure the client understands the following:

*   He or she will identify a discrete concern in step 1.
*   He or she will learn some self-hypnosis trance inductions from you during this session, to use in step 2.
*   Steps 3–6 are the steps that will take place during self-hypnosis; make sure the client understands how to fill out the template to plan these steps.
*   Step 7 is a reorientation step, in which to the client comes out of trance.

Teaching Self-Hypnosis

1. Guide the client through two or three self-hypnosis inductions for use in step 2. Choose ones you normally use in your practice or use the examples in the next section. Explain each method to the client in advance, maybe even demonstrating or role-playing it yourself.

2. For each method, guide the client through the steps of trance induction, remarking on the ease of the experience. You might want to remind your client that trance is a normal, everyday occurrence often experienced in moments of daydreaming, concentrating deeply, watching television, playing computer games, or when mentally rehearsing a conversation. You might also mention that in hypnosis one often encounters stray thoughts, and the way to handle those thoughts is simply to acknowledge them, thank them for being there, and then go back to the suggestions, plans, or visualizations.

3. Reassure the client that he or she can replicate what takes place during this session and practice self-hypnosis at home.

4. Tell the client to close his or her eyes (or just focus on some object in the room, gazing intently at it), relax, concentrate on some internal representation for a few moments (perhaps a pleasant memory), and then "return to conscious awareness." Say, "The experience you just had is similar to what happens in trance."

5. Guide the client through two or three self-hypnosis inductions (see the examples that follow), so the client can choose the one he or she likes the best. For each one, gently guide the client into trance, ask the client to imag-

ine a pleasant setting or remember a pleasant event, and then reorient. Then ask about his or her comfort and understanding of the process. Example:

How was that for you? Do you have any questions about the process? Is there anything that we could change that would make it better for you? Are you ready to do it on your own, or do you want me to guide you through it again?

6. For each type of self-hypnosis induction, let the client practice the induction and reorientation without help. Obtain feedback and answer questions. When the client has practiced two or three methods, ask which one he or she is most comfortable with. Then spend the remainder of the session helping the client practice that one and commit it to memory.

Just in case you need some extra help with teaching trance induction, the following are some standard self-hypnosis methods and a sample script for each one.

Self-Hypnosis Inductions

These three time-tested methods of hypnotic trance induction can be used to teach self-hypnosis. For each one, the client should be seated comfortably. Explain each one and guide the client through it, using the following scripts as examples of what to say. After each induction, ask the client for any questions or concerns. Allow the client to practice each induction more than once, to develop familiarity with the process.

Thumb and Index Finger Induction

This method was taught by Kay Thompson (Kane and Olness 2004). In it, the client pinches the thumb and index finger together as an anchor for going into trance.

Take your thumb and index finger and pinch them together tightly. You can close your eyes if you wish. Take a deep breath. Hold it as I count from 1 to 5 ... 1, 2, 3, 4, 5. Let go and bring those fingers apart. Feel a sense of relaxation as your fingers release. Take three more deep breaths now, and with each breath, give your full attention to your body. Notice its comfort and relaxation. It's almost as though you are going down into this more profound, comfortable kind of state. And when you get to that third deep breath, you are at the level where you can talk to yourself—the way you do when you are at home or any other appropriate place where you want to focus attention on your own thoughts.

At that point, you might say to yourself, "As I relax and focus my attention, I pay attention to the things I say to myself." And then talk to yourself about and mentally rehearse those things that are important to your outcomes. An appropriate suggestion you can give yourself now is that at any time in the future when you are in a safe, quiet place when you pinch your thumb and index finger together, and take that deep breath and let it out, that will be a signal to your subconscious mind to devote attention to this ability to go into trance and listen to yourself and focus on your goals. Your abilities will improve with practice. And after you do that, and your subconscious mind knows that it knows all it needs to know, you take another couple of deep breaths and emerge from that trance, 5–4–3–2–1, opening your eyes and feeling alert once more.

Arm Levitation Induction

For this induction, I sit directly in front of the client and demonstrate what I am asking him or her to do.

Sit comfortably, with your elbows loosely at your sides; bend your arms at the elbow and dangle your hands over your lap. Let your hands bend at the wrist, so that your fingertips are just barely touching your lap. Let your hands feel loose and limp.

Now do just as I do, so that you can anticipate how arm levitation feels. Slowly lift your right arm, bending it at the elbow, so that your hand seems to float up gently, away from your lap. As your hand and arm begin to lift, take a deep breath, closing your eyes if you wish, and relax. You might wish to lower your chin slightly. Your arm will stop rising several inches above your lap, almost at the level of your shoulder. Enjoy a sense of relaxation. ... Now lower your arm and hand slowly back down to your lap, and when your fingertips touch your lap, lift your chin, and open your eyes.

Repeat the process with your left arm. Slowly lift your left arm so that your hand floats gently up and away from your lap. Continue slowly to lift your arm up to shoulder level. Take a deep breath, and close your eyes if you wish. Relax for a moment. Again, enjoy the relaxation. ... Now lower your arm and hand slowly back down to your lap, and when your fingertips touch your lap, open your eyes.

Now stop demonstrating and continue to sit in front of the client, with your hands resting in your lap. Guide the client through the process, using the following script. Say words such as "lift," "lifting," "up," and "lighter" on the client's inhalation so that he or she will notice the sensation of lightness that naturally accompanies expansion of the chest. Modify the script as needed to match your observations of the client.

Having practiced this movement, you are now ready to discover how easily you can use it as a signal that you are going into trance. Keeping your elbows loosely at your sides, bending your arms at the elbows, and sitting comfortably, let your wrists bend so that your fingers are barely touching your lap. Stare at the space between your hands.

Become curious ... wondering which hand your subconscious mind is choosing for you ... choosing that hand to lift up ... as that hand begins to feel slightly different from the other one. You might begin to feel a slight sensation. Perhaps one hand begins to feel lighter—or perhaps you notice some small movement as one hand and arm are just about to lift. That hand and arm begin to lift ever so slightly now, making small movements, floating up now, as your subconscious shows you in a very handy way how cooperatively it responds to your every thought.

Your hand and arm float up effortlessly, guided by your subconscious mind. As your hand continues to rest at the end of your wrist, you can take a deep breath and relax, even closing your eyes if you wish. And while you are relaxing in this way, you might be aware of how easy it is to enter into this trance, and how easily you could use this comfortable state to talk to yourself about those things you want to accomplish in terms of your eating patterns, or things you want to motivate yourself to do regularly—those things you want to be conscientious about.

Remember that you can use this easy method of self-hypnosis at any appropriate time and place. Simply seat yourself comfortably in a quiet place, free of distractions, let your fingertips dangle on your lap, and concentrate on the space between your hands, allowing your subconscious mind to lift one hand for you while you drift into a hypnotic state to concentrate on outcomes and solutions, to strengthen your resolve, and to access your resources.

Then, as now, when a few moments have passed, slowly lower your hand to your lap at the same rate and pace as you open your eyes and return to full alertness, feeling refreshed.

Eye-Fixation Induction

This method and its variations have been used extensively in hypnotherapy. The idea is to instruct the client to fix his or her gaze on some object above eye level, so that the muscles around the eyes begin to feel fatigued. When the client takes a deep breath and closes the eyes, there is a sense of relaxation as the muscle strain around the eyes is released. This version is an adaptation based on the work of Michael Yapko (1990):

As you listen to the sound of my voice, lift your eyes toward the ceiling and search for some spot to look at—find something of particular interest to you. When you find that spot, continue to stare at it. Notice every detail of the way it looks. Keep looking at it, and as you continue to relax, notice how tired your eyes have become. And as your eyes grow more tired, your eyelids become heavier and heavier, and soon you want to blink. As you continue to blink, your eyes want to close. So take a deep breath in and hold it. Then, as you lower your gaze, close your eyes on the exhale, and feel a wave of relaxation come over your body as you relax more comfortably in your chair.

Optional eye closure: I ask you to relax your eyelids so much that they don't even want to open. You can pretend they feel so heavy, you don't even want to make the effort to try to open them. Let your eyelids relax so much that they just won't open. Try to open them and find you don't want to. And when that happens, it's a signal that you are in a hypnotic state and ready to access the resources within your mind in some remarkable ways.

As you continue to enjoy this state of relaxed concentration, you can take this opportunity to talk to yourself and focus on those changes you are making and those things you want to do differently to accomplish your ideal weight. Each time you practice self-hypnosis in this way, or any other way, you become more skilled. When you are ready to end your self-hypnosis, simply sit up, take a deep breath, open your eyes, and look around, feeling alert and refreshed, as I am asking you to do now.

Wrap-up

1. Now that you have taught your client at least one method of trance induction for self-hypnosis, guide the client through the Seven-Step Self-Hypnosis process, using the method of induction the client chose.

2. Help the client complete the self-hypnosis template, or use one of the sample templates in the *Client Workbook,* if one seems appropriate.

3. Show the client that the assignment also contains a self-hypnosis script for making an audio recording at home, using the seven steps. Encourage the client to spend a few minutes each day practicing self-hypnosis at home.

Client assignment for session 3: Give the client the take-home assignment for session 3: "Learning Self-Hypnosis," on the *Client Workbook* CD. The client should practice self-hypnosis a few minutes each day until the next session.

Self-Hypnosis Template

Step 1: Problem or concern: _____

_____

Step 2: Self-Hypnosis Induction: Take a deep breath and focus your concentration.

Step 3: Create the solution: how you want to respond differently—how you will think, act, and feel.

New thinking:

_____

_____

New feeling:

_____

_____

New actions:

_____

_____

Step 4: Visualize yourself carrying out the solution in a situation that previously would have been challenging. This is your mental rehearsal.

_____

_____

_____

_____

_____

Step 5: Your positive affirmations:

_____

_____

_____

_____

Step 6: Your posthypnotic suggestion:

From now on whenever I encounter

_____

I _____

_____

_____

Step 7: Reorient yourself: Open your eyes, stretch, and take a deep breath. Done!

Practitioner Checklist and Notes

Session 3: Training in Self-Hypnosis

Copy, complete, and put in the client's file.

Checklist	Notes
Client's name: _____ Date of session: _____ ❏ Follow up on any questions or concerns from the previous session on the Six-Step Reframe. ❏ Briefly discuss the previous take-home assignment: "Trim-Slim Thinking versus Fat Thinking" from the *Client Workbook*. ❏ Go over this session's home assignment: Learning Self-Hypnosis, and teach the client the Seven-Step Self-Hypnosis process. ❏ Demonstrate a few different methods of trance induction and allow the client to pick whichever is most comfortable for him or her. ❏ Have the client practice one method of trance induction for self-hypnosis until he or she feels confident in performing it. ❏ Give the *Client Workbook* assignment for Session 3: "Learning Self-Hypnosis," and tell the client to practice self-hypnosis sessions at home for a few minutes daily.	

Chapter 9

Session 4: Stopping Emotional Eating with Stress Management

Purpose

Many people overeat as a response to emotions, not true hunger. Many of my clients have told me that they overeat mainly when they are under stress. This all-too-common problem suggests the need for stress management skills. The purpose of this session is to teach clients how to manage stress, using NLP (for anchoring a resourceful state), so that they are less likely to turn to food as an antidote to difficult emotions.

Procedure

1. Ask the client for feedback regarding the previous session, then for a progress report on self-hypnosis.

2. Ask about any improvements in eating habits and weight management. Respond to any questions or concerns.

3. Explain that the purpose of this session is to reduce the client's tendency to overeat in response to stress or unhappiness, not by finding substitute activities for overeating (as in session 2), but by learning how to manage emotions and thoughts by changing them.

Educating Your Client That Emotions Can Be Changed

Not all clients will come to you with the understanding that many emotions, or mind-body states, can be changed. Some will have the attitude, "Well, that's just the way I feel, and I can't do anything to change it." These clients will benefit from some education on how to change emotional states. Here is a sample script with some things you might want to say.

> Do you have emotions, or do your emotions have you? That's the question. Until now, when you felt uncomfortable emotions or felt stressed out, you soothed your emotions by finding something to eat—maybe something fattening. Some people have a certain "comfort food" that they turn to when they feel upset or lonely or angry. Now, you know you can do other

things to soothe yourself, instead of eating. You might, for example, listen to some favorite music or take a walk or soak in a hot bubble bath.

The problem with using food as an antidote for emotions is that when you look at the end result of all that overeating, that just leads to more stress. What you have tried to do with "emotional eating" is to change an uncomfortable emotional state, or at least reduce its intensity. Humans seem to have a built-in rule that uncomfortable emotions are not to be tolerated for very long. Taking some action often seems to help reduce the emotional intensity in the short run, but the end result may not be healthy. Today, you'll learn how you can change your emotions in other ways, so that distressing emotions don't even show up.

I wonder if it sounds strange to you to say that you can change your emotions at will—that you can design your own emotional states. Instead of feeling nervous at a business meeting, you could feel calm. Instead of feeling scared about delivering that sales presentation, you could feel confident. Instead of feeling tired and anxious when you get home at night, you could feel relaxed and carefree, looking forward to the evening.

This may sound impossible, but it isn't. Our emotions are based on our impressions of the world around us, the associations we make by noticing similarities, and the meanings we attach to events. What if you made other associations and attached different meanings to everyday events? What if you could access more resourceful states in response to events that previously seemed stressful and troublesome? That's what you'll learn to do today, through an NLP technique called "anchoring." It helps you "anchor" yourself in resourceful mind-body states so that you are no longer adrift on a sea of distressing emotions.

Anchoring a Resourceful State

The following template shows the steps in helping your client learn to anchor a resourceful state. Where applicable, a sample script has been included.

Prior to beginning this process, watch the client's eye accessing patterns, to determine where (to the right or left of the visual field) the client accesses past and future. Most people access the future on the right side of the body and the past on the left. You'll be using skills in well-formed outcomes (the criteria are listed in step 2) as well as in the processes of calibration, anchoring, and future rehearsal.

1. **Get an example of the problem.** Ask the client to describe a recent experience of turning to food as a coping mechanism to soothe emotions or stress.

   Tell me about a time recently when you felt stressed out or unhappy in some way and you got something to eat—maybe some comfort food—not because you were hungry, but because you were trying to calm down those emotions. Give me a specific example: what was going on, where it happened, what you were doing, what you thought about, and what you felt, up until the moment you decided to get something to eat.

Once the client has described the example, ask him or her to go back, in memory, to that moment and access the thoughts and feelings. Note the "trigger," or specific stimulus, that launched the client into distress. Calibrate the client's breathing, facial expression, and posture, so that you can actually see the client's state of distress. Then bring the client's attention back to the present moment, sitting with you in your office. Help the client to interrupt and dismiss any remaining feelings of distress. In NLP this method of interrupting a state is called "creating a break state." It can be accomplished by changing the topic of conversation, by asking the client to change position, or by some other distraction. Say, "Okay, put all those emotions aside [Make a hand gesture to the client's left, as though moving all those feelings to the client's past.] and be here now with me."

2. **Obtain a well-formed outcome and a congruent commitment to change.** Ask the client, "In the future, when that kind of situation arises, what response would you rather have? How do you want to think and feel differently?" [Gesture to the client's future and encourage the client to look up in that direction.] "How do you see yourself behaving differently?"

   Make sure the client describes a well-formed outcome that meets these criteria:
   • is stated in the positive (avoids "I will not ...")
   • concerns future actions (versus regrets about the past)
   • is self-initiated and self-maintained
   • is specific and observable
   • is realistic
   • is stated without equivocation
   • is ecologically sound.

3. **Help the client access and anchor a resourceful state.** Ask the client to identify an internal resource, that is, a resourceful state or a way of feeling, that would permit the envisioned change to occur. Then ask the client for an example of when he or she has experienced that resourceful state. *The context for the resourceful state should be entirely unrelated to the problem context.* If the client's resource is "confident," for example, ask for a context in which the client reliably feels confident. In the following sample dialogue, "confidence" is used as an example of an auditory anchor. It's best to use the client's own word for the resourceful state. Say the word, using the client's inflection and tonality, in order to pace the client's experience and reinforce the anchor word.

Ask the client to re-create the context in memory and revivify the resourceful state:

Be there now, feeling confident. [Apply the auditory anchor.] Remember what you saw and heard, what you were doing at that moment, what you thought and how you felt. Recall all those confident feelings and have them again.

Bring the client back to the present moment and check to make sure the resourceful state the client remembered is uncontaminated, satisfying, and suitable as a replacement for the client's previous problem state. If the remembered resource state does not meet these criteria, have the client experiment with other remembered resourceful moments in order to find a state that is a good "fit" as a resourceful state.

Having found a suitable resourceful state, guide the client back into the memory.

Be there now, feeling confident again. Remember what you are seeing, what you are hearing, and what you are doing, thinking, and feeling. Recall all those confident feelings and have them again. [Apply the anchor.] This time, hold on to those feelings and memorize them. Own them, so that you can take them with you, and you can have those confident feelings whenever you want them, now and in the future. Your anchor word for these feelings is "confidence." Whenever you say "confidence" to yourself, or I say "confidence" to you, you reaccess those feelings of confidence. The cue will bring back those confident feelings so that you become accustomed to having confidence whenever and wherever you want it.

Now come back to the here and now with me, bringing all that confidence with you.

4. **Overlay the anchored response onto the problem state.** Ask the client to reaccess the problem context identified in step 1, but this time in response to the "trigger," apply the anchor and tell the client to imagine the same situation, only feeling much more resourceful. Invite the client to have a different result, and to notice the difference.

Now that you have a reliable method for accessing confidence, take yourself back to the problem situation you told me about earlier. Everything is as it was before, as you remember it, except this time as that same _____ [Describe the trigger.] occurs, you feel confidence. Notice what happens now. Discover a change for the better when you access confidence. When you notice what has changed, bring your attention back to the here and now with me, and tell me about it.

Ask the client to describe what was different in the pseudo-remembered scenario, when he or she applied the resource anchor. Evaluate the change. Repeat this step three to five times to condition the new response. Make sure the client is satisfied with the new response. If not, choose another anchor to "stack" on top of the first anchor. Address any ecological concerns as they arise.

5. **Future rehearsal.** Have the client imagine future instances in the "real world" that are similar to the problem context and where he or she wants to respond with the resource state instead of the old problem state. Guide the client through mental rehearsals in which he or she mentally rehearses applying the anchor to access a resourceful response. Ask the client to report on a few of these, on what he or she imagines. Praise the client for learning a new response, pointing out that this is a new way of handling stress *"so that you have a new way to respond to those types of situations that were previously difficult, but now are much easier to manage."*

6. **Reinforcement with hypnosis.** Now use a brief hypnotic induction to review and reinforce everything you have taught the client in this session. Use the following script or make up your own.

Brief Script to Reinforce Coping Skills

As you continue to review and plan the changes *you are making changes today,* consider that you have in your possession all the learning and understandings … acquired over a lifetime, to support *you … are managing how you feel, what you think, what you decide, and what you do.* As you subtract old patterns that no longer serve you, you multiply your coping skills and define your qualities, inner wisdom, intuition, and inner strength in new ways while *you have solved those previous problems,* and realize *you can easily distinguish between true, actual hunger and emotional distress.*

Increasingly, *you see new options and possibilities* while *you nurture yourself* by deciding what to notice and what to ignore, what to hold on to and what to let go of, and when to say yes and when to say no. You are worth it. I recommend that *you approach the world increasingly on your own terms, and according to your values and beliefs, progressively finding congruity and integrity and personal satisfaction by coming from a place of inner honesty, confidence, self-caring, and peace beyond measure.*

Your _____ [Name the client's resource here.] *is growing stronger each day,* as you find additional contexts and situations where you are applying that _____ [resource]. Your mind is like a toolbox and your _____ [resource] is a tool like, say, a screwdriver. Maybe it's nice to discover you can use it for many more tasks than just tightening a screw to keep something in place. You can, for example, use it for prying a container open to get at the contents inside, or for getting something unstuck so that it works more smoothly and effectively.

Now and frequently, when you think about all the times when *you are successfully applying your* _____ [resource] *in various situations,* you might notice how *you are doing it effectively* and what is the one change that makes all the difference—that secret success factor that makes it work. *You now increasingly refine that success and integrate it into your thinking on a daily basis as a means of strengthening your coping skills as you acquire all the self-assurance that you now have available,* and use it as your new response to those situations that were so difficult before but now seem much more manageable. Sometimes food for thought is all you need to feel better.

Appreciate yourself for what you are learning, and the improvements you are making, as you open your eyes, once more feeling quite alert.

Client's assignment for session 4: Give the client the take-home assignment for session 4: "Stress Management and Emotional Eating" on the *Client Workbook* CD. Remind the client to reduce four pounds (or two kilos) in order to attend the next session.

Practitioner Checklist and Notes

Session 4: Stopping Emotional Eating with Stress Management

Copy, complete, and put in the client's file.

Checklist	Notes
Client's name: _____ Date of session: _____ ❑ Follow up on any questions or concerns from the previous session or the at-home assignment on self-hypnosis. ❑ Help the client anchor a resourceful state for coping with a stressful situation. ❑ Help the client apply that resourceful state to other similar situations. ❑ Give the *Client Workbook* assignment for session 4: "Stress Management and Emotional Eating." ❑ *Remind the client to reduce his or her weight by at least four pounds (two kilos) in order to attend the next session.*	

Chapter 10

Session 5: Making Sensible Food Choices

Purpose

The purpose of this session is to apply hypnotherapy to motivate the client to choose healthful, nutritious, low-calorie foods over fattening foods.

Procedure

1. Congratulate the client on having lost the required weight to return for this session and ask what strategies helped with weight reduction. Follow up on the previous session and ask what changes the client is noticing in managing stress, and whether this has made a difference with "emotional eating."

2. Talk to your client about the importance of good nutrition and eating a balance of
    *   fruits and vegetables
    *   complex carbohydrates such as whole grains
    *   lean meats (unless your client is a vegetarian)
    *   non-meat proteins such as legumes, lentils, and nuts
    *   dairy products
    *   healthy fats such as olive oil, flaxseed oil, and omega-3 fatty acids
    *   water

    Modify the items on this list if your client has food allergies or dietary restrictions affecting any of these food groups. Ascertain your client's outcome for this session by asking what foods he or she considers healthful and nutritious, and what foods he or she wants to avoid or eat only in small quantities. The underlying theme for this session is to make distinctions and use those distinctions to make wise choices about what to eat. Ask your client what suggestions he or she would like to hear in today's hypnotherapy session that would encourage healthy, sensible choices about food.

3. Prepare to audio-record this session. Make sure your client is seated or reclining comfortably and is ready to listen. Record the following script,

adding suggestions the client would like to hear and adapting the script to the client's needs and preferences. Remember to stress the words in italics. As you read through this script, insert deepening instructions as needed.

Hypnotic Script for Sensible Food Choices

Induction and Reassurances[6]

A good way to begin is to make sure *you are comfortable.* ... And, with eyes closed ... scan your body to notice where you'd like to get a bit more comfortable or relaxed ... where you could send soothing thoughts and feelings of contentment ... until *you feel so relaxed,* you are ready to have a rewarding hypnotic experience, in which *you are amazed at how effectively ... your mind and body are responding at many levels ... to ensure ... you are making wise, empowered choices about food.*

To *relax more completely* ... take a long, slow, deep breath, and as you release that breath, let it be a reminder ... that the ability to breathe deeply ... and to observe deep breathing can be an asset ... in managing stress ... *feeling calm and confident ... making decisions ... and thinking clearly.*

So breathe in deeply and slowly ... and just as slowly exhale ... while you *focus your mind ... to create new discoveries.* Breathing freely and easily ... just letting go of distractions ... so that you truly experience and enjoy the moment ... the present ... a gift you give to yourself ... breath after breath ... *relaxing more comfortably ... twice as deeply.* ... Each moment flows into the next moment ... moment after moment ... as motivation acquires momentum ... and confidence and self-assurance become stronger ... guided by your inner wisdom ... finding mementos along the way ... an evolving vision of yourself ... moment after moment ... breath after breath.

Now, whether or not you are familiar with the experience of hypnosis ... I hope you understand that it is your own, personal experience ... an experience you create for yourself ... unique for each individual. You can, _____, [Insert client's name.] ... *be in a deep hypnotic state now* ... yet you remain aware of your surroundings. ... Or you might have an intense inward focus ... to the extent that my voice fades in and out. ... Or perhaps you forget to listen at the conscious level ... while *your subconscious mind becomes more attentive.* ... Or you might be aware that ... *you are drifting into a soothing, deep, peaceful state ... with the relaxation enveloping your mind and body with each breath you exhale ... so calm ... so quiet ... so much more comfortable than moments before.*

While ... *you are relaxing now,* here are some things to remember, for your comfort, safety, and satisfaction with this hypnosis experience. No matter *how deeply ... you are relaxed,* you are free to move about to become even more comfortable. You can open your eyes and end this process at any time you desire and for any reason you desire. While you are listening to this recording, should anything occur that requires your immediate attention, you will instantly return to full alertness, open your eyes, move about, and attend to the matter without delay.

So for now you can simply ease back and enjoy the experience, with the understanding that hypnosis is an opportunity *to empower your motivation, access your inner strength and knowledge ... and see additional possibilities.* So, no matter ... *how deeply ... you are relaxed ... you are free to accept or reject anything I say.* If I say something that isn't helpful or relevant ... your mind will automatically dismiss it and ignore it. It will have no negative effect whatsoever.

... To the same extent, when I say *suggestions that are useful and helpful, then I trust ... your inner mind will absorb these ideas and recommendations ... integrating them with your beliefs and values, altering perceptions and understandings so that ... desirable changes are becoming evident ... in your thinking, feeling, and acting ... in ways that are healthy and positive ... so that in the days and weeks to follow ... you are experiencing benefits and improvements ... physically ... mentally ... and emotionally,* so that it is absolutely true you are making wise choices about food.

As you prepare to *explore this hypnotic state more completely,* I invite you to begin *now* ... to make some distinctions and notice some differences: ... the difference between when we were talking moments ago and what it is to just listen now ... without having to say or do anything for a while ... the difference between expecting to *relax* ... and actually *allowing that relaxation to occur.* ... Perhaps you notice that your breathing has slowed ever so slightly ... as your physical activity level slows ... allowing your muscles to relax with ease. Perhaps your thoughts are less active, too ... as you are concentrating on the words I say ... or developing your own solutions. ... Less concerned about the environment around you ... and more concerned about the inner world of mind ... and thoughts and ideas ... and awareness of those things most relevant to your intentions.

Perhaps you agree that the ability to notice differences and make distinctions is the basis of making choices. ... Just as you can choose to relax a little, or *relax very deeply.* ... You might feel cooperative, or merely curious. ... You might choose to *absorb this information* at the conscious level ... or just *rely on your subconscious mind to take it all in and produce satisfying results.*

Change Work

This ability to make choices really means *you take control* ... because you can choose this or that. ... And because you can choose, you can be choosy. ... Interesting, isn't it? Being choosy allows for making distinctions. ... Sometimes you have no choice but to be choosy ... when the alternative to being choosy is something you would never choose. ... When people choose to be choosy ... they have a way of knowing what they find acceptable and worthwhile. ... They *notice the differences between* quality and mediocrity, *what is a waste that goes to your waist, and between what is tasteful and what has no taste* ... what is important and what is trivial ... what is enduring and what is temporary ... *what foods are nutritious and what foods are fattening.* ... After all, everyone can *recognize the differences* between a pear and a pastry, a bran muffin and a brownie, a glass of wine and a glass of water, a carrot and a candy, and you do, don't you?

Sometimes choosiness changes over time. ... The things you might have chosen before are not always those you would choose today ... *because your sense of taste can change, and some things don't taste as good as they once did, and some things taste better* ... and good taste never goes to waste.

When you are choosy about what you read, it's because *you care about what you feed your mind.* ... If you are selective about the music you listen to and the kinds of television shows and movies you watch, *it's a matter of preference, aesthetics, and personal taste.* ... Maybe it's the way you furnish your house or the colors you like or the kinds of people with whom you associate that shows ... *you have a sense of quality. What you put into your body really matters because it makes a difference.*

Just as charity begins at home, *finding contentment begins with loving yourself*—even loving your body. Which car would you rather ride around in? An old, rusty clunker that guzzles gas, oozes oil, moans and groans, stalls out in the fast lane, and can't pass a safety inspection, or a reliable, sleek, sporty car?

It's just one more reminder that, _____, [Insert client's name.] once you make up your mind, you can *do what you set your mind to* ... without ever minding what your mind thought would be difficult. Foregoing an unhealthful food sometimes really turns out to be a blessing in disguise ... because your mind and body begin to mind what you say ... and you can finally have your say ... *while the choosiness makes you more mindful than before.* No amount of fattening food is as satisfying as *finding increasing delight in those feelings of self-confidence and accomplishment when you choose foods that are healthful and non-fattening.*[7]

The truth always rings true and resonates throughout the spirit. So when you consider which foods to eat and which foods to avoid, I don't need to tell you what a trance-formation occurs when *you eat only healthful foods* ... and *you feel fed up with fattening foods.* ... Choosiness is a challenge, yet this change is the chance to *make healthful choices* ... while challenging old haphazard habits of not being choosy at all ... when choosy is better than chubby.

Healthful foods are _____. [List foods that are healthful for your client, such as fresh fruits, vegetables, salads, lean meats, whole grains, beans and lentils, and low-calorie snacks.] Consider the tangy, tart sweetness of a strawberry or a juicy orange as you bite into it and the taste floods your mouth. Who could possibly resist the satisfying crunch of a crisp cucumber or an apple? Plump, ripe tomatoes are tangy and almost bursting with a succulent taste that speaks of country roads and farms and warm summer days and nostalgia. Peaches and pears taste like the melodies of springtime. Cooked beans and lentils summon up the warmth of home and hearth, and clear soups and broths might remind you of staying cozy on a cold day. Nature nurtures through her bounty of nutrition.

Trust that your subconscious mind provides you with sufficient inner guidance to shop intelligently, plan your meals carefully, and choose nutritious, healthful foods ... such that you are experiencing a glow of delicious, luscious satisfaction as those extra pounds disappear in the sweet pleasure of honoring and respecting your body's needs ... in accordance with your glowing passion to feel and look and be healthy and attractive at the weight you choose to achieve and maintain. _____ [Here, add any suggestions your client has selected.]

It would be interesting, I think, to bottle self-awareness, discipline, and tenacity ... and put them into a pill or a potion that people could just purchase ... in a store or by mail or by e-mail ... so anyone could reduce their proportions. No need to push a pill with such a pull *that you automatically enjoy nutritious and healthful, slenderizing food in ways that astonish you and delight you.*

Posthypnotic Suggestions and Future Rehearsal

I suppose you'll digest all this for a while ... about noticing differences ... making distinctions ... having choices and how to, _____, [Insert client's name.] *exercise choice about the foods you eat ... and how to slim down to that lasting, favorite weight* ... making up your conscious mind ... and *your subconscious mind,* and not even noticing at first that ... *you are already using this information effectively* ... and what it means to you ... *while you choose your own conclusions.* When you weigh the options and consider the choices, *you create astonishing results and do so consistently* ... so that the changes you make are lasting and permanent— for as long as you wish.

I don't know whether *the changes you are making* ... are taking place gradually or quickly, or all at once or incrementally. ... I only know that you have the capacity to *achieve the results you choose* in ways that are positive, pleasant, and healthful for you.

Reinforcement

I recommend that each time you listen to this recording ... *the positive suggestions are more effective and powerful* ... enhancing your progress. ... *The changes in your thought patterns and behaviors* ... *more productive and satisfying as you are increasingly attracted to low-fat, low-calorie, healthful, nutritious foods that are tasty and slenderizing.*

Ending and Reorientation

If you are listening to this recording at night in bed, and you wish to go on to sleep, you can simply keep on relaxing, moving into a healthy, restorative sleep. I wish you lovely dreams that *amplify all positive suggestions*, and suggest that you wake up refreshed in the morning. If you wish to drift into sleep, just ignore the following instructions. [Pause about ten seconds before continuing.]

On the other hand, if you are listening to this recording during the day and wish to return to the day's activities, [Pick up the tempo of your voice here.] give me your attention because now it's time to become fully alert again. Feel yourself become more alert, coming up now, feeling more energized, ready to return to conscious, wakeful awareness, fully alert now, eyes open, feeling fine. [Make sure the client is fully alert.]

Wrap-up

Stop recording and ask the client to take a quiet moment to think back over the session. Ask about any questions or concerns that might have surfaced and address those issues.

Client's assignment for session 5: Give the client the take-home assignment for session 5: "A Two-Week Food Diary," on the *Client Workbook* CD. Remind the client to reduce at least four pounds (or two kilos) as a requirement for attending the next session.

Practitioner Checklist and Notes

Session 5: Making Sensible Food Choices

Copy, complete, and put in the client's file.

Checklist	Notes
Client's name: _____ Date of session: _____ ❑ Ask about the client's success in reducing four pounds (two kilos) since the previous session. ❑ Follow up on any questions or concerns from the previous session on stress management. ❑ Answer any questions about the previous session's at-home assignment "Stress Management and Emotional Eating" in the *Client Workbook*. ❑ Conduct and audio-record the hypnotherapy session focusing on healthy food choices. ❑ Give the completed recording to the client. ❑ Give the client a copy of the assignment for session 5: "A Two-Week Food Diary" from the *Client Workbook*. ❑ *Remind the client to reduce his or her weight by at least four pounds (two kilos) in order to attend the next session.*	

Chapter 11

Session 6: Creating an Intelligent Relationship with Food

Purpose

The purpose of this session is to apply hypnotherapy to motivate the client to develop intelligent decision making about when to eat, how to eat, and when to stop eating. The message here is, "Tune in to your body's messages and sensations, so that you eat only when you are hungry and stop eating when you are full, and feel satisfied and happy with yourself for doing so."

Procedure

1. Ask about the client's weight reduction since the previous session. What factors contributed to the client's success in reducing by at least four pounds (two kilos)? What was easy or difficult? What worked well and what didn't work so well? Commend the client's efforts. Give encouragement for the next four pounds (two kilos) he or she will reduce.

2. Follow up on the previous session and ask what changes the client is noticing in selecting healthful foods and beverages and avoiding or limiting fattening foods and beverages that are high in sugar, salt, fat, cholesterol, and alcohol. Inquire about the client's problems or successes in completing the two-week food diary assignment. Answer any questions and encourage the client to articulate what he or she learned from the assignment.

    Some clients will report that the assignment was a hassle or an inconvenience, which is understandable since it requires keeping track of food choices and being consciously aware of caloric intake—something people who are overweight don't do very often. Empathize with and explore the client's feelings about being more aware of calories and what kinds of foods he or she selects. If the client is having trouble understanding which foods are healthy and which are fattening, or has trouble counting calories, give any practical advice you can and direct the client to additional sources of information (Internet web sites, nutritional books and pamphlets, a local nutritionist, or classes on nutrition).

3. Ask your client what suggestions he or she would like to hear in today's hypnotherapy session in order to encourage an intelligent relationship with food, defined as eating when hungry and stopping eating at the point of feeling full. The underlying theme for this session is enhanced body awareness—tuning in to sensations of hunger and satiety.

4. Prepare to audio-record this session. Make sure your client is seated or reclining comfortably and is ready to listen. Record the following script, adding suggestions the client would like to hear and adapting the script to the client's needs and preferences. Remember to stress the words in italics. As you read through this script, insert deepening instructions as needed.

Hypnotic Script for Creating an Intelligent Relationship with Food

Induction and Reassurances

To *relax your mind and body* ... and focus your thoughts, ... close your eyes ... and consider all that you are aware of at this moment ... *the sound of my voice* ... perhaps other sounds as well, sounds in the room ... sounds outside the room ... aware of the space around you ... the surface on which ... *you are relaxing—more deeply now.* ... *Aware of your breathing—perhaps you'd like to count your breaths as I speak, until you feel so relaxed, you need not count anymore.*

Hold out your arm and imagine ... you are holding in that hand the handle of a bucket of sand ... and *feel that weight—every ounce of it—a very heavy burden ... much too heavy ... uncomfortably heavy ... weighting you down.* Getting more and more annoying ... burdensome ... all that weight ... and yet what are you weighting for? The ordeal of having supported that weight ... thinking to yourself it wasn't so bad ... trying to put up with it ... *yet, it gets more burdensome by the moment.* ... *You feel so intensely ... the desire to release it ... to lower that weight ... to be relieved of it ...* and holding on to all that weight has proven more difficult and tiring. ... The strain, the discomfort ... as you are now finding a way to weigh the weight that you were waiting to weigh ... while you realize ... the heavy weight was just too much to tolerate ... so heavy that you could not possibly ignore it ... a discomfort ... causing you now to get a handle on things ... reaching out for the solution and holding on to it. ... And while you lower your appetite and raise your expectations ... you began to release that burden now and lower your hand ... lower that weight ... lower that weight, more and more. As your hand goes down, you drift more deeply into the experience ... and your subconscious mind multiplies your motivation to have the weight you choose.[8]

So you are free of that heavy weight ... the sand in the bucket, the sand in an hourglass—time passing ... life passing by ... time doesn't wait ... *refusing to wait any longer ... to have the weight you choose ... finding the way ... the method ... the path ... the direction ...* and following it with pleasure and relief ... happy to advance to a more complete hypnotic state.

While ... *you are relaxing now,* here are some things to remember, for your comfort, safety, and satisfaction with this hypnosis experience. No matter *how deeply ... you are relaxed,* you are free to move about to become even more comfortable. You can open your eyes and end this process at any time you desire and for any reason you desire. While you are listening to this recording, should anything occur that requires your immediate attention, you will instantly return to full alertness, open your eyes, move about, and attend to the matter without delay.

And for now, you can attend to the moment. ... Moment by moment ... each moment continues to the next. ... Time passes ... all the time you need in such a short time ... to find the consistency that wasn't there before ... yet available to you all along ... strengths and resources ... tapping into them ... in moments of contemplation and reflection ... automatically ... within the mind, ... where all is known ... while you feel safe and secure ... there ... while I speak to you here ... as you access the power of your mind.

As *your perceptions become more internally focused* ... perhaps *more aware than before of those internal indications from the body ... subtle variations in pressure ... fullness ... energy level, ... heartbeat, ... internal sounds, ... vibrations, and rhythms ... that tell you so much—when you feel warm and want to cool down ... when you feel tired and ready to rest ... when your stomach is empty and you turn to nourishment ... when your stomach is full and you stop eating. Let your subconscious mind guide you* ... as you learn to ... *trust your body more. ... Let it guide you ... into an intelligent relationship with food.*

No matter ... *how deeply ... you are relaxed ... you are free to accept or reject anything I say.* If I say something that isn't helpful or relevant ... your mind will automatically dismiss it and ignore it. It will have no negative effect whatsoever. ... To the same extent, when I say *suggestions that are useful and helpful,* then I trust ... *your inner mind will absorb these ideas and recommendations ... integrating them with your beliefs and values, altering perceptions and understandings so that ... desirable changes are becoming evident ... in your thinking, feeling, and acting ... in ways that are healthy and positive ... so that in the days and weeks to follow ... you are experiencing benefits and improvements ... physically ... mentally ... and emotionally.*

Change Work[9]

There are ways of thinking about food that you may find helpful as ... *you reach your favorite weight and size in a timely manner* ... with the fullness of understanding that you have the resources you need to *make these suggestions work for you in powerful ways.* ... Getting what you choose is not about willpower or deprivation. ... They don't work. ... What works is to, _____, [Insert client's name.] *end the senseless struggle with food—and define the power of your intelligence to understand and attend to and respond to your body's messages.*

Eating is a natural, enjoyable human activity. ... Food is nourishment, and hunger is the body's request for nourishment. When you were eating not for nourishment, but for relief or for comfort—you missed out on the enjoyment of food.

To have an intelligent relationship with food, understand that it's okay to eat. ... You can eat whatever and whenever you want ... as long as *you eat slowly and place your full attention on every bite ... so that you really enjoy the food itself. ... By eating mindfully in this ... weigh ... less ... is more satisfying, because* you derive more satisfaction from food so you eat less food. ... When you concentrate on every bite ... time ... slows ... down ... so that the simple process of eating a sandwich ... can feel like eating a full-course meal. ... As you acquire this new way of eating, *your preferences have already begun to change. ...* When *you eat slowly and mindfully,* and with full attention to every bite ... you discover the freedom to choose when and where and what to eat for nourishment.

Therefore I recommend, _____, [Insert client's name.] you eat when you can devote your full attention to eating. ... Eating one bite at a time. ... If you are eating a meal ... you put your fork down after every other bite and pause. ... Take a deep breath and feel relaxed ... aware of the sensations of eating and digesting. Eating in this manner, you find that half of what you ate previously is sufficient to satisfy your nutritional needs. ... And yet you feel full and satisfied with just the exact amount of food that maintains the body weight you choose, when you are look-ing and feeling healthy, trim, and fit.[10]

Form an image in your mind of your appearance … exactly the way your body looks when you are maintaining your favorite size. … A rich, focused image, programming your mind and body so that you pursue this outcome with clarity of thought and action … and your conscious mind and your subconscious mind agree to bring that image into reality. … Your focus and consis-tency are stronger now … so that you no longer resist having it … and you give in over and over again to the overpowering temptation to have the body size and shape you desire.

As that yearning and determination grow stronger, your mind makes lasting changes that sat-isfy you, while your subconscious mind is collecting memories of times and places where you are *dealing with food in an intelligent, competent manner,* [Pause about ten seconds.] and those memories form a lasting learning that stays with you.

In the meantime, allow *your subconscious mind to make a shift, … slowly taking your ability to burn those calories and turning it up, so that … while you remain healthy … those fat cells are getting smaller … and that extra fat is disappearing under the energy of a super-charged metabolism. …* At the same time, *your subconscious mind readjusts your understandings and perceptions in such a way that when you encounter fatty, greasy, sugary foods … your sub-conscious mind sends a powerful, commanding, compelling message throughout your body that says, "No, _____."* [Insert client's name.] And that no resonates so that the no … N – O … actually enhances what *you* know you know, and instead of life revolving around what to eat or not to eat, it becomes much more comfortable to *make healthy decisions … as your pleas-ure with life increases proportionately.*

As these changes take place … you feel a sense of satisfied self-confidence … while review-ing those things you do competently and confidently … your skills and talents. … In fact, imag-ine you are performing one of those activities now … feeling skilled … feeling competent. Be there now, in that moment, doing something at which you are very skilled and competent. See the surroundings, hear the sounds … feel the movements … think the thoughts … have the same feeling of confidence now as then. … [Pause about ten seconds.] *Capture those feelings of satisfied self-confidence and memorize them … so that you can apply those same feelings in other circumstances where they are useful … you can feel them right now and every time … you are making thoughtful and competent decisions about food. …* And that satisfied self-confidence can intensify to the extent that … *every intelligent choice feels wonderful for you.* … This is how to create good feelings for yourself and enjoy those feelings more each day.

Next, remember a time of feeling so full you could not eat another bite. … Be there again now. … Remember how it feels … feeling so full that you cannot eat another bite. [Pause about ten seconds.] … Let your body memorize that full, full feeling, so that … *from now on, you have that feeling—so full you cannot eat another bite—whenever you should end your meal or snack. … Thus, when you begin a meal or a snack, your conscious mind and unconscious mind can agree on the exact right amount to eat. … And when you have eaten that exact right amount … eating slowly and consciously … then you feel so full you cannot eat another bite. … And when you have made that intelligent decision … once more, you enjoy that feeling of satisfied self-confidence.*

You might like to discover how you feel when … *you trust your body enough again to tune in to those subtle communications … exploring that quiet sense of self-awareness … eating only when you feel hungry … choosing nutritious foods … stopping when you feel full … and feel-ing good about yourself the entire time.*

Posthypnotic Suggestions and Future Rehearsal

Moving your thoughts to the future … *you practice making wise choices about food* … at restaurants, at parties and picnics, at work, and at home. Enjoying success, day after day, … until eventually, you find you've made an unwise choice … but you get right back on track again with smart choices. … Then, a few days later, again another poor choice, but *you just have that much more determination to get right back on track again with smart choices.* … Observe that even while you make occasional unwise choices about food … *you are shedding those excess pounds* the entire time. … Now you have the secret! … *Getting the weight you choose* is not about perfection. … It's about *persistence* … realizing *that every setback is an opportunity to get back on track with smart choices*—and each time that full, satisfied self-confidence feels so good … *it is worth doing again and again.*

Reinforcement

I recommend that each time you listen to this recording, *the positive suggestions are more effective and powerful* … enhancing your progress. *The changes in your thought patterns and behaviors … more productive and satisfying.*

Ending and Reorientation

If you are listening to this recording at night in bed, and you wish to go on to sleep, you can simply keep on relaxing, moving into a healthy, restorative sleep. I wish you lovely dreams that *amplify all positive suggestions,* and suggest that you wake up refreshed in the morning. If you wish to drift into sleep, just ignore the following instructions. [Pause about ten seconds before continuing.]

On the other hand, if you are listening to this recording during the day and wish to return to the day's activities, [Pick up the tempo of your voice here.] give me your attention because now it's time to become fully alert again. Feel yourself become more alert, coming up now, feeling more energized, ready to return to conscious, wakeful awareness, fully alert now, eyes open, feeling fine. [Make sure the client is fully alert.]

Wrap-up

Stop recording and ask the client to take a quiet moment to think back over the session. Ask about any questions or concerns that might have surfaced and address those issues.

Client's assignment for session 6: Give the client the take-home assignment for session 6: "The NLP Slender Eating Strategy" on the *Client Workbook* CD. (This material is duplicated in appendix I for quick reference.) Remind the client to reduce four pounds (two kilos) in order to attend the next session.

Practitioner Checklist and Notes

Session 6: Creating an Intelligent Relationship with Food

Copy, complete, and put in the client's file.

Checklist	Notes
Client's name: _____ Date of session: _____ ❑ Ask about the client's success in reducing four pounds (two kilos) since the previous session. ❑ Follow up on any questions or concerns from the previous session. ❑ Discuss the previous session's at-home assignment: "A Two-Week Food Diary" in the *Client Workbook*. ❑ Conduct and audio-record the hypnotherapy session that focuses on eating when hungry and stopping eating when full. ❑ Give the completed recording to the client. ❑ Give the *Client Workbook* assignment for Session 6: "The NLP Slender Eating Strategy." ❑ *Remind the client to reduce his or her weight by at least four pounds (two kilos) in order to attend the next session.*	

Chapter 12

Session 7: Boosting Motivation to Exercise

Purpose

The purpose of this session is to apply hypnotherapy to motivate the client to exercise regularly in a safe and healthy manner. The underlying theme for this session is enhanced motivation. A word of caution for this session: Make sure that the client has chosen a form of exercise that is safe, healthy, realistic, and in accordance with his or her health, time-management, and financial circumstances.

The script for this session was developed specifically for clients who dislike exercising—which seems to be the case for most people with weight issues whom I've met. The suggestions are generally appropriate for "polarity responders"; that is, independent thinkers who resist being told what to do, even when they know the recommendations are in their best interests. Polarity responders tend to unconsciously dig in their heels and block themselves from obtaining their stated outcomes because of an underlying drive to "be my own person" or "decide for myself."

Many obese clients don't like exercise because they associate exercise with past coercion from gym teachers, drill sergeants, or sports coaches. I have had some clients who associate physical activity with having to "perform" for someone else. One woman told me that she hates to go for walks or to the health spa because she feels self-conscious and conspicuous exercising in front of other people. Some people who are overweight dislike exercise because of joint pain or the exhaustion they feel upon the slightest exertion. Due to these considerations, the script uses "reverse psychology," which "prescribes the symptom," suggesting that the client will try to resist the attraction of exercise and eventually give in to it.

Note: Ask the client what types of exercise he or she wants to undertake. Use what you know about physical activity and elicit information from the client to create a vivid description of that particular activity. The following script has a place to insert that description. The description should include the visual, auditory, and kinesthetic aspects of that exercise, and verbs should be in the present tense. Include the values that the client attaches to exercise, such as grace, coordination, muscle tone, increased energy and stamina, attractive appearance, strength, and so on.

Procedure

1. Ask how the client was successful in reducing by at least four pounds (two kilos) since the previous session. What factors contributed to the client's success? What was easy or difficult? What worked well and what didn't work so well? Commend the client's efforts. Encourage the client to continue reducing the next four pounds (two kilos).

2. Follow up on the previous session and ask what changes the client is noticing in terms of eating when hungry and stopping when full. Ask about any problems or successes the client had with the "NLP Slender Eating Strategy" assignment in the *Client Workbook* (also in appendix I). Answer any questions and encourage the client to articulate what he or she learned from the assignment.

3. Prepare to audio-record this session. Make sure your client is seated or reclining comfortably and is ready to listen. Record the script, adding suggestions the client would like to hear and adapting the script to the client's needs and preferences. Remember to stress the words in italics. As you read through this script, insert deepening instructions as needed.

Hypnotic Script for Motivation to Exercise

Induction and Reassurances

To begin ... perhaps you'd like to remember times in the past when you've felt relaxed. ... Play back memories of entranced concentration. ... *Consider carefree relaxation ... comfortable, restful times ... soothing carefree moments ... when time passes unnoticed ... a pleasant restfulness of hands and feet ... arms and legs ... a trance-formation of awareness ... an alignment of mind and body ... how easy it is to feel so aware ... of your own ability to allow deep relaxation to occur. ... And the mind relaxes the body ... the body relaxes the mind, and so on ... as your subconscious mind becomes more attentive ... accepting responsibility for guiding ... and directing ... and the relaxation deepens while you remember that you really possess the ability to relax,* to allow the mind to be totally unconcerned about how or why ... or even about making the effort to try to understand ... and instead *allowing a process of learning and discovery to take place at multiple levels of intelligence and intuition ... while you simply relax ... the mind ... the body ... quiet and peaceful ... where all that matters are the words, your intention ... your experience ... and the presence and the presents of your own inner wisdom ... gifts to yourself.*

While ... *you are relaxing now,* here are some things to remember, for your comfort, safety, and satisfaction with this hypnosis experience. No matter *how deeply ... you are relaxed,* you are free to move about to become even more comfortable. You can open your eyes and end this process at any time you desire and for any reason you desire. While you are listening to this tape, should anything occur that requires your immediate attention, you will instantly return to full alertness, open your eyes, move about, and attend to the matter without delay.

As you relax even more, your breathing slows. Your heartbeat slows to a steady, even pace. A steady pace brings progress toward your outcomes as you learn to sustain momentum moment by moment … directing your attention and energies where they matter. … Movement matters … motivation, momentum. Movement … getting into shape … shaping the future of your body … less weight is more freedom.

And no matter … *how deeply … you are relaxed, you are free to accept or reject anything I say.* If I say something that isn't helpful or relevant … your mind will automatically dismiss it and ignore it. It will have no negative effect whatsoever. … To the same extent, when I say *suggestions that are useful and helpful,* then I trust … *your inner mind will absorb these ideas and recommendations, … integrating them with your beliefs and values, altering perceptions and understandings so that … desirable changes are becoming evident … in your thinking, feeling, and acting … in ways that are healthy and positive … so that in the days and weeks to follow … you are experiencing benefits and improvements … physically … mentally … and emotionally.*

Change Work

As *you get more comfortable* … it's easier to understand how energy creates activity and activity creates energy … and the more energy you use … the more energy you have. … So let's examine this business *about exercise … because you choose to exercise* … but you didn't like it … but you want the results … but you had other things to do … but you choose to reduce your weight. … *So you move that but* around … *and it takes on a new shape* … and things change. … And your mind knows what matters when it's mind over matter … or is it matter over mind? … Or does it really matter? … When *what matters is allowing your mind and body to function as though your body matters* as much as your mind.

After all, you have a conscious mind and … *you have a subconscious mind* … and you have a right brain and a left brain. … What matters is to *use the right mind* when it's right to use the right one, and it's right to use the left one when the left one is the right one. … *It wouldn't be right if you left exercise out of your formula for success.* … What matters is how you know what's right for you to use for what really matters. … Your right cannot be your left, but your left can be right, when *it's the right choice,* and sometimes *the right choice is the only choice left for you* to make it *work out* right.

I wonder whether you desire to exercise excessively or moderately, based on moderately excessive desire. After all, when it comes to your physical well-being … no one can *make up your mind* for you. … No one really knows what it takes to *convince yourself to have the full enjoyment of it.* … Not everyone is smart enough to *make up your mind and do it.* … You think for yourself … not like some weakling who sits around and whines about being out of shape until people *refuse to listen to the excuses.*

In the past, perhaps you resisted the urge to exercise—having put forth feeble, non-motivating thoughts and then felt disappointed with those weak, halfhearted efforts that didn't, _____, [Insert client's name.] *work out with abandon and joy.* Maybe you've heard it said … disappointment comes from doing everything but the right thing … which is the only thing left to do that really will … *work out.* … And what works out is *whatever it takes to exercise* common sense.

I could say to you, "_____, [Insert client's name.] *just do it! Stop dawdling and come to terms with it. Get off the bench and into the game. Get off your seat and move … butt."* … It's

101

not my decision. ... The secret to life mastery is the ability to form an outcome ... *decide to do it ... believe in yourself ... make a real commitment ... put your passion into it, and take consistent action ... and feel that sense of integrity and self-satisfaction ... that lifts the spirit as well as the metabolism.*

I ought to tell you the story of a fat old dog I once had ... who liked nothing better than to lounge around the house ... like an old dowager. ... The vet said, "She needs *exercise!*" ... But she disdained my invitations to go for walks. ... If I scolded her, she would only go hide under the bed. ... So I coaxed her with enthusiasm: *"Come on! Yes! Come on! You can do it! Let's go! Let's go! Let's get moving! Come on! It will feel great!"* ... And sure enough, she would *get up and go!* ... *Sometimes eagerly, sometimes hesitantly, but doing it regardless.*

Therefore, you could simply continue to ... *exert all the effort you can ... powerfully and gracefully ...* to resist that overpowering urge to exercise ... because the more you try in vain to resist it ... *the stronger the compulsion to do it becomes. ... Even distractions and inconveniences make it so much more compelling ... you become obsessed with the joy of exercising.* ... Still, try to avoid the inevitable satisfaction ... until *you are convinced ... you just refuse to sit still ...* for the disappointment you might have felt with previous attempts.

As you try unsuccessfully to resist the overpowering desire to exercise ... you find *you are continuously thinking about exercise—wishing for it, longing for it, wanting to sneak some in—*but hold on and get firm, trying without success to ignore those constant thoughts ... and find *you cannot not exercise.* This *resistance becomes a heavy burden to lug around* ... but keep trying until ... *nothing can stop you* when *you make up your own mind—the most powerful creation in the universe—*to apply in any way. ... You *see fit ... ness comes with the price of pure pleasure with your body ...* and only you can decide when *you are ready, willing, and eager to move forward into that activity.*

_____ [Here, insert the vivid V-A-K description of the client's chosen form of exercise.]

So you realize the answer is ... at hand ... when for some people the right hand is right, and for some the left hand is right, and sometimes the other hand can become the right hand with which to write ... *the understandings you need ...* while making this change becomes as right as putting one foot in front of the other ... and taking the next step and making the next move. ... When you do ... it's easy to remember how difficult it was at first ... to say yes or no, which is your right ... and you're left with the right choice ... *when you understand you have a right to exercise your right to have your right weight ... without waiting around ... but getting right to it ... so you weigh less and you feel better ... stronger ... more energized.*

Posthypnotic Suggestions and Future Rehearsal

Imagine looking into the shiny, iridescent crystal ball of the future and seeing what awaits you— what you've been wishing and waiting for—come to life—an image of you ... feeling *active and healthy—*with that heart-pounding excitement, *strong and fit, capable and confident. ... You are comfortable with your body and comfortable in your body ... comfortable moving your body.* ... Now you grasp the possibilities realistically and intelligently ... moving, bending, and stretching ... breathing hard and sweating ... as you muscle your way into a new comfort zone called feeling healthy.

Imagine how it is to enjoy movement and strength ... to explore your physical capacities for agility, flexibility, speed, power, or grace. ... To bend and stretch, and push and pull and lift, and flex and extend. ... To feel your heart beating and your pulse pumping, and to breathe hard and heavy, and to sweat. ... To know what it is to go the distance. ... You are entitled to the satisfying, gratifying, well-worth-it, tired feeling of flushed, warm contentment that arrives after vigorous and safe physical exertion.

Exercise your right to a healthy body. ... Find the athlete ... the warrior ... the jock ... the wild one within ... who yearns to *express your physical vitality and energy. Break out of those bonds of sedentary lethargy* ... and *celebrate the body in motion* ... as life takes on a new rhythm ... a routine ... a steady, reliable persistence ... both reassuring and invigorating—*feeling the vitality that rejuvenates you.* ... New ideas *take shape attractively ... based on a burning desire ... like an engine burns fuel to generate energy ... like a love affair with yourself.* ... Exercise is not a sacrifice—it's a healing ritual, a sacred communion ... a celebration of what your body can do and the way you take care of it as you would any prized possession—with respect and reverence.

Reinforcement

I recommend each time you listen to this recording ... *the positive suggestions are more effective and powerful* ... enhancing your progress. ... *The changes in your thought patterns and behaviors* ... *more productive and satisfying. Each time you listen to this tape, your subconscious mind is more responsive ... taking in the suggestions more completely.*

Ending and Reorientation

If you are listening to this recording at night in bed ... and you wish to go on to sleep, you can simply keep on relaxing, moving into a healthy, restorative sleep. I wish you lovely dreams to *amplify all positive suggestions,* and suggest you wake up refreshed in the morning. If you wish to drift into sleep, just ignore the following instructions. [Pause about ten seconds before continuing.]

On the other hand, if you are listening to this recording during the day and wish to return to the day's activities, [Pick up the tempo of your voice here.] give me your attention because now it's time to become fully alert again. Feel yourself becoming more alert, coming up now, feeling more energized, ready to return to conscious, wakeful awareness, fully alert now, eyes open, feeling fine. [Make sure the client is fully alert.]

Wrap-up

Stop recording and ask the client to take a quiet moment to think back over the trance experience, perhaps even closing his or her eyes to review what occurred. Ask the client about any questions or concerns that might have surfaced and address them.

Client's assignment for session 7: For this session's at-home assignment, the client will read the report entitled "The Benefits of Exercise" on the *Client Workbook* CD (also found in appendix J for quick reference) and complete the assignment for session 7: "Mind Management." Remind the client to bring the "Mind Management" assignment back for session 8, because the affirmations and words of encouragement from that assignment will be incorporated into the script for session 8. Remind the client to reduce his or her weight by four pounds (or two kilos) in order to attend the next session.

Practitioner Checklist and Notes

Session 7: Boosting Motivation to Exercise

Copy, complete, and put in the client's file.

Checklist	Notes
Client's name: _____ Date of session: _____ ❑ Ask about the client's success in reducing four pounds (two kilos) since the previous session. ❑ Follow up on any questions or concerns from the previous session. ❑ Discuss the previous session's at-home assignment: "The NLP Slender Eating Strategy" in the *Client Workbook*. ❑ Conduct and audio-record the hypnotherapy session focusing on motivation to exercise. ❑ Give the completed recording to the client. ❑ Tell the client to read "The Benefits of Exercise" and complete the assignment for session 7: "Mind Management," both in the *Client Workbook*. ❑ *Remind the client to reduce his or her weight by at least four pounds (or two kilos) in order to attend the next session.*	

Chapter 13

Session 8: Pulling It All Together for Lasting Results

Purpose

The purpose of this session is to apply hypnotherapy to reiterate the client's original outcomes, incorporate affirmations, and suggest lasting outcomes. The themes for this session are self-affirmation, self-acceptance, and lasting success.

Procedure

1. Ask about the client's weight reduction since the previous session. What factors contributed to the client's success in reducing by at least four pounds (two kilos)? What was easy or difficult? What worked well and what didn't work so well? Commend the client's efforts and encourage him or her to continue working to reach the target weight.

2. Follow up on the previous session. Did the client read the "Benefits of Exercise" report? Inquire how the client is doing with developing or maintaining an exercise routine. Emphasize that long-lasting success at weight reduction is much more likely with regular exercise. Respond to any questions or concerns the client may have.

3. In preparation for this session, the client should have read and completed the take-home assignment for session 7: "Mind Management." Briefly discuss the assignment and review the affirmations and specific messages of encouragement and suggestions the client has chosen for today's session. Additionally, review your Practitioner Notes from the previous seven sessions for any helpful suggestions or reminders you can incorporate into the script for this session. You will see places in the script to insert the client's affirmations, words of encouragement, and other helpful reminders about outcomes, insights, and discoveries.

4. Prepare to audio-record this session. Make sure your client is seated or reclining comfortably and is ready to listen. Record the following script, adding suggestions the client would like to hear and adapting the script to the client's needs and preferences. Remember to stress the words in italics. As you read through this script, insert deepening instructions as needed.

Hypnotic Script for Pulling It All Together

Induction and Reassurances

Make yourself as comfortable as you like ... taking a long, deep breath ... perhaps closing your eyes and ... drifting into a peaceful, calm state ... where mind and body work together ... where logic meets intuition ... creativity blends with intellect ... desire merges with fulfillment ... and decision creates conscientious, consistent action. ... Potential becomes possibility becomes reality when you realize ... how much more completely ... *you can focus your thoughts and feel relaxed and at ease* ... already beginning, perhaps to, _____, [Insert client's name.] *have a satisfying experience of hypnosis in which you are amazed ... at the changes taking place at multiple levels ... levels of mind ... levels of physiology ... even the functioning of your neurology conforms to your image of yourself at your chosen size.*

Every cell in the body receives the essence of every thought ... every belief ... everything you tell yourself ... through neurological communication channels. ... Every system in your body has its own intelligence ... and the conscious mind and subconscious mind fulfill many functions ... mentally, physically, and emotionally.

While ... *you are relaxing now,* here are some things to remember, for your comfort, safety, and satisfaction with this hypnosis experience. No matter *how deeply ... you are relaxed,* you are free to move about to become even more comfortable. You can open your eyes and end this process at any time you desire and for any reason you desire. While you are listening to this recording, should anything occur that requires your immediate attention, you will instantly return to full alertness, open your eyes, move about, and attend to the matter without delay.

No matter how deeply ... you are relaxed, you are free to accept or reject anything I say. If I say something that isn't helpful or relevant ... your mind will automatically dismiss it and ignore it. It will have no negative effect whatsoever. ... To the same extent, when I say *suggestions that are useful and helpful,* then I trust ... *your inner mind will absorb these ideas and recommendations ... integrating them with your beliefs and values, altering perceptions and understandings so that ... desirable changes are becoming evident ... in your thinking, feeling, and acting ... in ways that are healthy and positive ... so that in the days and weeks to follow ... you are experiencing benefits and improvements ... physically ... mentally ... and emotionally.*

Prepare to *relax so deeply now that your thoughts guide you to discover unexplored potential and claim the treasures awaiting you. ... Along the way, access your creativity, your intuition, your inner wisdom as you create remarkable, lasting changes at many levels.*

Change Work

When you consider unhappy events of the past ... and the emotions that didn't digest well ... the things you didn't know then that you know now ... you might enjoy the changes occurring *in that master control system that empowers you to manage eating, metabolism, energy, and appetite sensibly and astutely. ...* And it's possible to remember now that ... *your body is precious ... a delight ... a joy ...* remembering now how to ... *attend to its natural mechanisms of communication ... tapping into innate knowledge ... offered freely by this remarkably intelligent, complex, sophisticated system of mind and body. Your subconscious mind is rearranging things ... in accordance with circumstances that are different now.*

As you, _____, [Insert client's name.] *remove from your mind any associations ... inhibitions ... disappointments ... fears ... distractions ... anything that ever influenced you to overeat. ... Now that you have freed your mind from unnecessary attachments to food ... what*

106

did being overweight say for you that you now say for yourself? ... *You don't have to carry around extra weight to find an abundance of love and goodness in yourself.* ... What is the void you avoided filling with happiness? ... *When you fulfill your life ... not with food but with self-esteem ... so you love yourself, you love your body ... discovering how much more you delight in treasuring your personality, your mind, and your body.*

I wonder whether ... you can *visualize a soft, glowing glimmer of healing light*[11] ... shimmering with beautiful colors ... soft and nurturing ... comforting ... beginning at your heart center—a healing presence of love and reconciliation. ... A light gently pulsating and expanding ... a light bringing delight and lightening your burden. ... *The light represents the consciousness of your spirit and inner strength—a dynamic, healing force.* ... *I don't know exactly what colors are in the light,* ... *or whether it is warm or cool.* ... *Yet, having just the softest intensity ... it is guided by an intelligence to know exactly where and how ... to focus the energy ... to heal ... to correct ... to adjust ... an energy beginning to circulate throughout your body ... gently and softly ... reaching into every molecule ... imparting wisdom and knowledge to every cell.* ... *Infusing every tissue ... in a very safe and selective way ... cleansing and shining into ... every organ and every structure of your being ... altering your physiology and cognitions ... such that all your healthy outcomes are manifesting ... bringing your ideal weight into reality ... refining your appetite ... balancing your energies ... shifting your capacity for healthy, joyful living.*

The restorative glow is flowing through your neurological system ... bringing *welcome changes in understandings and perceptions that seem miraculous and remarkable ... and at times so subtle you hardly notice them ... lest you think they are too good to be true ... too true to be few ... as you become accustomed to new sensations ... new size and shape ... new vitality and pleasure, and the satisfaction of recognizing the differences ... and meeting the challenges with confidence.* ... *You develop a more profound sense of self ... fulfilled.*

There are things more important than food ... a larger sense of life purpose and passion. ... *Imagine loving your body ... without needing food to feel loved ... to discover how lovely it is to be you, inside and out.*

Perhaps you have a sense of this light now ... with its special colors ... beaming with love and compassion ... yet so calming and relaxing. ... *Enhancing self-worth and self-acceptance—feeling comfortable in your own skin.* ... *Feeling forgiveness for past situations that are over and done, while you embrace your strengths ... and appreciate your finer qualities, ... shining forth your best version of* _____ . [Insert client's name.]

Imagine, visualize, or feel this healing light moving *through every fiber of your being.* ... Maybe it sounds like music ... perhaps a symphony or a lullaby ... as it courses through your bloodstream and your neurology ... and into organs and tissues ... joints and bones ... into every cell glowing with life and vitality ... bringing a message of *loving yourself, caring about your body ... your health ... your energy ... finding peace and contentment in being you.*

Resolving the negative experiences of the past ... is similar to watching an old, grainy black-and-white movie of those events ... and a younger version of you then ... from across the expanse of time and space ... running the movie fast forward and then fast backward ... and fast forward ... and fast backward ... and fast forward ... and fast backward ... so many times ... that the movie blurs ... the memories become lackluster ... and fade into trance-lucent obscurity, *and you are free to take your place in among confident ... healthy individuals ... meeting challenges with flexibility, logic, clear thinking ... intelligence, adaptability, and a philosophical equanimity ... based deep within a conviction and confirmation of the spirit of wisdom ... beyond comprehension and peaceful determination ... beyond mere wishing ... as your comfort with loving who you are increases ... finding those occasional moments of inexplicable contentment ... as it pleases you to do so.*

The light gives you *a sense of your own power to navigate and negotiate the difficulties of life ... your own ability to protect yourself ... and look after your own best interests ... a knack for solving problems and seeing safe, viable opportunities and possibilities. ... The light surrounds you with love and stays with you ... the glow of being you.*

You have allowed me to repeat the following affirmations, suggestions, and recommendations.

_____ [Here, insert the client's affirmations from the "Mind Management" take-home assignment. State these affirmations in second person (using "you," as in "You are a caring, loving, lovable person").]

Now as I repeat these affirmations, say them to yourself along with me.

_____ [This time, insert the client's affirmations, in first person (using "I," as in "I am a caring, loving, lovable person").]

_____, [Insert client's name.] you have also given me permission to say to you the following words of support and encouragement: _____ [Here, read the words of encouragement the client has listed as part of the "Mind Management" take-home assignment.]

Here are additional suggestions and recommendations: _____ [Here, insert any other suggestions or recommendations you have written in your notes from previous sessions.]

Posthypnotic Suggestions and Future Rehearsal

As you continue to enjoy many changes in your life ... I congratulate you and commend you for your courage and your progress ... in achieving and maintaining the weight you choose ... the body size you choose ... trim and healthy ... because you are implementing these guidelines ... consistently, reliably, successfully.

As you venture forward, day by day ... you will meet temptations to overeat or exercise less ... you might take small excursions off the familiar path ... yet you keep going ... because each detour brings you back on course with healthy eating patterns and regular exercise. ... You meet difficulty with improved coping skills. ... As you become healthier, your self-confidence increases ... you are firm but gentle with yourself ... a coach and friend ... a trusted advisor. ... You discover you can manage and resolve discomfort ... without turning to food ... and you are solving problems more effectively ... responding to challenges more resourcefully and skillfully.

From now on, when you look at old photos of yourself when you were overweight, two words are etched indelibly in your mind. ... Never again ... never again ... never again. ... As you travel along your timeline into each future present ... each present future moment ... presents to you ... these opportunities to operate reliably and effectively ... and you treasure the pleasure of feeling healthy and fit ... and many sweet discoveries along the journey.

Reinforcement

I recommend ... each time you listen to this recording ... *the positive suggestions are more effective and powerful* ... enhancing your progress. ... The changes in your thought patterns and behaviors ... more productive and satisfying.

Ending and Reorientation

If you are listening to this recording at night in bed, and you wish to go on to sleep … you can simply keep on relaxing, moving into a healthy, restorative sleep. … I wish you lovely dreams to *amplify all positive suggestions* … and suggest you wake up refreshed in the morning. … If you wish to drift into sleep, just ignore the following instructions. [Pause about ten seconds before continuing.]

On the other hand, if you are listening to this recording during the day and wish to return to the day's activities, [Pick up the tempo of your voice here.] give me your attention because now it's time to become fully alert again. Feel yourself become more alert, coming up now, feeling more energized, ready to return to conscious, wakeful awareness, fully alert now, eyes open, feeling fine. [Make sure the client is fully alert.]

Wrap-up

Stop recording and ask the client to take a quiet moment to think back over the trance experience, perhaps even closing his or her eyes to review what occurred. Ask the client about any questions or concerns that might have surfaced and address them.

At the end of this session, give the client your recommendations, including suggestions for additional therapy sessions with you, if appropriate. See chapter 18 for suggestions of follow-up sessions that may be of benefit. Also consider referrals to other health-care practitioners and services, and to information sources such as web sites, books, CDs, DVDs, classes, seminars, and conferences. If the client does not want follow-up sessions, provide information about your future availability, in the event the client wants your services at a later date.

Say your farewells and offer the client your wishes for success. I recommend you plan to contact the client in three months with a follow-up phone call or e-mail, to check on progress and offer any additional sessions that might be helpful.

Client's assignment for session 8: Give the client the take-home assignment for session 8: "Keep Going: Make Changes Last, Make Motivation Last" on the *Client Workbook* CD.

Practitioner Checklist and Notes

Session 8:Pulling It All Together for Lasting Results

Copy, complete, and put in the client's file.

Checklist	Notes
Client's name: _____ Date of session: _____ ❑ Ask about the client's success in reducing four pounds (two kilos) since the previous session. ❑ Follow up on any questions or concerns from the previous session. ❑ Discuss the previous session's at-home assignments: "The Benefits of Exercise" report and "Mind Management" worksheet. ❑ Ask the client what affirmations and words of encouragement to incorporate into this session's script. These will come from the "Mind Management" assignment. ❑ Conduct and audio-record the hypnotherapy session, focusing on the theme of lasting changes. ❑ Give the completed recording to the client. ❑ Give the *Client Workbook* assignment for session 8: "Keep Going: Make Changes Last, Make Motivation Last." ❑ Discuss recommendations for any future appointments, resources or referrals to other professionals.	

Chapter 14

Additional Session:
A General-Purpose Script

The following script is for an extra session. You can use this script in several ways:

- As a "booster" session for clients who are having trouble maintaining an exercise regimen and nutrition plan.

- As a substitute session when for some reason or another, one of the sessions 2 through 8 does not meet your client's needs. You might want a replacement session for a client who already knows self-hypnosis (session 3) or who can't think of a stress management issue (session 4) or who is already exercising routinely (session 7).

- As a follow-up session for clients who have completed the program but want to return later for support and reinforcement.

You may want to audio-record this session. When you present this script, adapt the wording to the sensitivities and preferences of your client. Be sure to stress the words and phrases in italics.

Induction and Reassurances
Use an induction method and the deepening methods of your choice, or consult appendix F: "Eighteen Ways to Induce and Deepen Hypnotic Trance."

> While ... *you are relaxing now,* here are some things to remember for your comfort, safety, and satisfaction with this hypnosis experience. No matter *how deeply ... you are relaxed*, you are free to move about to become even more comfortable. You can open your eyes and end this process at any time you desire and for any reason you desire. When you are listening to this recording, should anything occur that requires your immediate attention, you will instantly return to full alertness, open your eyes, move about, and attend to the matter without delay.
>
> *Your choice to do what you set out to do is what makes hypnosis effective* ... because it speaks to your capacity to ... *turn desire into reality.* ... Since you recognize hypnosis is an opportunity to ... *empower yourself,* you also realize you are free to accept or reject anything I say to you. ... In fact, if I say anything that is not helpful or relevant, your mind will automatically reject it and dismiss it ... and it will have no negative effect whatsoever. ... Now, here's the best part:

For those things I say to you that are helpful and useful ... your subconscious mind will automatically accept those suggestions ... absorbing them at every level ... integrating positive suggestions completely and seamlessly with your beliefs and values ... modifying understandings and perceptions ... creating significant changes in your thinking, your emotions, and your actions ... implementing those suggestions in healthy, appropriate ways ... so that you notice and enjoy healthy and positive benefits and improvements day by day ... mentally, emotionally, and physically.

Change Work

Treat yourself now to the pleasurable vision of looking at yourself in a full-length mirror and imagining ... the more attractive, healthier you is looking back at you ... having now reached your target weight. ... See that [she or he] wears clothing in your desired size. ... See that [she or he] moves more easily and gracefully. ... [She or he] smiles with the glow of accomplishment. Like Alice, who stepped through the looking glass into Wonderland ... *step into that image and imagine the wonder of living your life in a body size that makes you feel happy, healthy, comfortable, and confident.*

Now you know what you didn't know before. ... *You realize food is for nutrition and energy, and you choose healthful foods wisely. ... Now you derive comfort from your intelligence, talents, and problem-solving skills. You benefit from your capacity to nurture yourself and soothe yourself in positive, life-affirming ways. ... You enjoy exercise because the benefits of physical activity are essential to a balanced lifestyle. ... You realize that your body is a complex, miraculous treasure to be treated with care and respect ... You comprehend that a healthy, fit body is your birthright and a supreme joy. ... Now you realize that it's absolutely true that you can have the weight you choose.*

You choose this healthier weight like an order for merchandise ... received, processed, filled, confirmed, and delivered. ... You've chosen this body size in the same way you choose a stylish, flattering outfit for a special occasion. ... *Your life is a special occasion. ... It is the celebration of you ...* _____ [Insert client's name.] *of invincible spirit.*

You've put the fears of the past to rest and allowed your subconscious mind to take care of the rest. Because you have accomplishments in your life ... *you understand what it is to set a goal and reach it with unshakable, single-minded determination ... while your confidence and self-assurance continue to strengthen in all ways. ...* You have transcended discouragement and frustration. ... *You've broken through the barriers of self-sabotage. ...* You have moved beyond doubt and negative thinking ... beyond disappointment ... *to discover the true power of your mind, trusting your abilities ... believing in yourself ... because you know how to keep a commitment to yourself ... faithful to your vision. ... You understand how to make a wish come true.*

Yes, you had to resolve some issues, and come to terms with and wrap up some loose ends, but the process is worth it, and the results are wonderful. ... *Now you know how to use your mind to evaluate options, generate solutions, and carry out your own decisions with skill.*

You have traded excess pounds and fat for a trance-formed quality of life. ... No more wishing and hoping and yearning for the weight you wanted. ... No, none of that. ... *The enjoyment of feeling fit and healthy is so irresistible you feel compelled to give in to it ... consistently buoyed by the momentum of motivation telling you success is inevitable. ... Having and maintaining a healthy weight is natural.*

If this step through the looking glass is appealing to you, then continue relaxing more deeply into trance. As I count from 1 to 5, you continue evolving and developing this best vision of yourself.

One ... now you realize what is possible and achievable. ... Two ... *now you use the unlimited power of your mind to envision a result, create that result, and make it real and lasting.* ... Three ... you have reached the moment of truth and come to terms with your choices. ... Four ... *the force of your subconscious mind moves you forward.* ... As you relax more deeply now ... *the magic is in you—taking hold of your imagination and motivation—to accomplish your vision purposely, conscientiously, skillfully ... in the certainty of doing what it takes ... in the certainty that your subconscious mind supports you, directs you, and guides you, leaving nothing to whim, chance, weak excuses, or halfhearted efforts ... all removed ... all dismissed.* ... Five ... *your subconscious mind is completely responsive to all positive suggestions and concepts ... making helpful, orderly arrangements and creative modifications to patterns and habits ... in which neurology influences physiology ... and the body and mind coordinate in agreement.*

The reconciliation and resolution of inner conflicts are a relief ... in the pleasure of a conscience untroubled by regret or frustration ... *tranquil and serene in the pleasures of healthful living honestly with yourself—a deep, abiding, precious peace of mind; contentment of heart; and secure self-reliance.* ... Life has deeper meaning than those old worries about food and fat and calories. ... There is a more meaningful purpose to living than obsessing about food.

Now that you have stepped over the threshold of possibility ... through the looking glass of your own psychology ... *the images and impressions are imprinted on your deeper mind—taking delight in your own strength, resources, and consistency.*

Nice to acknowledge ... *you give yourself permission to enjoy fulfillment ... having the weight you choose ... loving and valuing yourself ... treasuring your body ... taking pleasure in healthy actions ... content with the authenticity of holding yourself accountable to yourself ... simply because you are worth it, and you have what it takes to accomplish it.*

After all, why not have a body as beautiful on the outside as you are on the inside? ... If you have ever pursued something worthwhile ... the planning, negotiating, reminding yourself, giving yourself encouragement ... then *you understand what to do and how to do it, and you smile patronizingly at the pathetic irrelevance of doing otherwise.*

Posthypnotic Suggestions and Future Rehearsal

Stepping back out now, on this side of the looking glass ... you find that sufficient reason to change ... directing and guiding your thoughts, emotions, and actions. ... You are resolute in holding on to that meaning that inevitably overrides lesser considerations ... in the most delicious manner possible ... having discovered that for which you were really hungering all along. ... Now you keep this image of a more fit, healthier you in mind. ... The image, the words, the concepts enhance your motivation. ... Taking care of yourself according to this plan improves your effectiveness in all you do. ... It is a luscious indulgence ... the pleasure of looking in that mirror and seeing the body size you choose ... and loving it and celebrating it, feeling astonished ... and delighted each day with the changes you've made in your life.

Reinforcement

I recommend that each time you listen to this tape ... *the positive suggestions are more effective and powerful ... enhancing your progress. ... The changes in your thought patterns and behaviors are ... more productive and satisfying.*

113

Ending and Reorientation

If you are listening to this tape at night in bed and wish to go on to sleep, you can simply keep on relaxing, moving into a healthy, restorative sleep. I wish you lovely dreams that *amplify all positive suggestions,* and suggest that you wake up refreshed in the morning. If you wish to drift into sleep, just ignore the following instructions. [Pause about ten seconds before continuing.]

On the other hand, if you are listening to this tape during the day and wish to return to the day's activities, [Pick up the tempo of your voice here.] give me your attention because now it's time to become fully alert again. Feel yourself become more alert, coming up now, feeling more energized, ready to return to conscious, wakeful awareness, fully alert now, eyes open, feeling fine. [Make sure the client is fully alert.]

Part III
Enhancing Success

Chapter 15

Coaching the Stuck Client

Working with clients who have excess weight has its challenges. I continue to learn and witness a great deal about the difficulties this population faces. One major issue is maintaining commitment and motivation. It's a common behavior pattern of overweight individuals to drop out and give up on weight reduction programs, even when they start to see real results! Weight reduction is difficult and takes perseverance and discipline. In addition, if the weight functions as a psychological protection factor for the client, losing weight can create some fear and anxiety. In this chapter, I tell you how to recognize when a client is stuck and provide three methods for coaching a stuck client to get back on track. This chapter also contains a section on working with clients who do not like to exercise and advice on when to make a referral. First, however, let me tell you about my own first nineteen clients. I share this information with you to give you a snapshot of what it's like to work with people who are overweight.

My First Nineteen Clients

While writing this book and still developing the WHY Program, I gathered statistics on nineteen clients who participated in hypnotherapy-assisted weight reduction through my practice from 2002 to 2004. The group consisted of five males and fourteen females, ranging in age from 33 to 66 years with an average age of 45 years. With the exception of three clients who wanted to reduce only 25 pounds, the remaining participants all had clinical obesity, reporting excess weights of 40 to 100 pounds. The average excess poundage for this group was 59 pounds. As I write this, I am currently working with one client who is 200 pounds overweight and another who is 150 pounds overweight.

Of the nineteen individuals, only nine actually completed all eight sessions, with the remaining ten completing from three to seven sessions. Two clients who completed the program returned for additional follow-up sessions. Although I sent surveys to all nineteen clients for more information, only two clients returned their surveys, so I did not obtain sufficient information to record average weight reduction outcomes. Clients who corresponded with me or followed up with me during the three years reported weight reductions ranging from 0 to 70 pounds.

The 50 percent dropout rate was mainly attributable to two categories of problems. One category was health issues. When individuals with obesity reach middle age, they encounter a host of health issues that curtail physical activity. Obesity seems to accelerate the aging process. The health problems in my client population included joint problems (two clients dropped out because they required knee surgery and a long rehabilitation period), heart and cardiovascular problems, hormonal imbalances, diabetes, polycystic ovarian syndrome, and high blood pressure. Bear in mind that these problems are often accompanied by depression, which contributes to lack of motivation and diminished persistence in maintaining a nutrition and exercise program.

The second category consisted of unexpected life stressors, such as a death in the family, a job change, financial problems, or marital discord that lowered the priority of weight management. Again, these life stressors were often accompanied by emotional upheaval and depression, which decreased motivation and often resulted in a return to compulsive eating.

For individuals who are overweight to complete any weight reduction program and reach their goal weight, it is essential that they maintain a sense of commitment and involvement. When I first developed the program, I mistakenly assumed that charging the fee in advance and having clients see incremental results would suffice to motivate them to stay in the program and benefit from it. This is not the case for many individuals who are obese, however; they need so much more. They need coaching, monitoring, and encouragement.

Keeping Clients on Track

Weight reduction is for many an onerous and difficult endeavor. Part of the reason many people who are obese or overweight fail at weight reduction is because achieving one's desired weight requires determined, sustained effort over a long period of time, and the progress is slow, incremental, and fraught with the possibility of setbacks. It's easy to understand that many people will start a weight reduction program but give up due to discouragement, depression, slow progress, or perhaps conflicted feelings about their weight. They get stuck.

Cancellations and no-shows are usually a sure sign that a client is stuck. If a client starts canceling appointments, or doesn't keep appointments, decide whether you are willing to put in extra effort to help this person succeed. If it doesn't seem likely that your efforts will get results, you could leave it up to the client to initiate the phone call for additional appointments. After all, you have been paid in full, whether or not the client returns to finish the program. On the other hand, every client who successfully completes the program is a walking testimonial for your services—so it may be in your interest to encourage reluctant clients to complete the program.

If you haven't heard from a client for a while, phone to inquire as to why the client has not kept or scheduled additional appointments. Do not scold or blame. Listen. Stay in rapport and respond empathetically. Give any practical advice you can. For example, if your client has run into unexpected health problems, refer to a physician or encourage the client to consult his or her regular physician. If your client is under unusual stress, offer an extra stress management session.

If your client seems unmotivated and ready to give up, you have an opportunity to coach him or her back on track. Professional life/success coaches help people navigate the process of change and accomplishment. Coaches guide their clients to focus on strengths, commit to outcomes, develop plans and strategies, access internal and external resources, and adhere to timetables. This chapter contains three coaching strategies to apply when a client is no longer moving forward. The first strategy, managing the itinerary of change, helps the client marshal the attitudes, desires, and problem-solving patterns that move people forward toward the results they plan. The second strategy is reframing failure as an element of success. The third strategy is inviting the client to commit to the next step by reaching an accountability agreement.

These strategies involve the client in making the assessments and decisions that will further progress. The central elements in these strategies are "chunking down," "chunking up," asking questions, and getting specificity in response.

Chunking down: Chunking down is an NLP term. It means taking a large process or undertaking and breaking it into small chunks so that accomplishing the process is less overwhelming. Chunking down makes it easier to figure out what to do next.

Chunking up: Chunking up is another NLP term. It means perceiving the outcome in the grander scheme of things, as part of a larger vision, purpose, or significant aspect of fulfillment. Chunking up makes the outcome meaningful and worth going for.

Asking questions: The art of asking questions lies at the heart of coaching. It is the chief mechanism through which coaches communicate with their clients. Questions invite the client to think in new ways, as well as to stay involved in the conversation and in planning the course of events. You'll find plenty of sample questions in this chapter.

Specificity: Specificity speaks to making plans real. It asks when, where, how, how often, how many, with whom, or to what degree. Specificity makes action items measurable and realistic and facilitates accountability.

Managing the Itinerary of Change

When a client is stuck, it may be useful to determine where in the change process he or she has stalled. Then, with a series of questions, you can help the client get back on track with renewed commitment. In their book *Mastering Mentoring and Coaching with Emotional Intelligence*, trainers Patrick Merlevede and David Bridoux (2003) address the elements involved in successfully completing a long-term project and bringing it to completion. They propose that successful project outcomes follow an "itinerary of change," a sequence of decision points at which progress either continues or comes to a halt. The secrets for continuing progress are that the individual must have a compelling intention to accomplish the outcome, perceive the next step, believe the next step is possible, develop a strategy to overcome perceived obstacles, take action, and sustain action.

The sequence of the itinerary of change echoes the "do what it takes" philosophy so essential to the success of any significant endeavor. The structure of the chainlike sequence is desire → intend → want → can → allow → decide/choose → put in motion → sustain the effort → complete. Notice that each link in the chain is expressed as a verb—something the individual *does*. Let's examine the sequence in more detail:

Desire: People who accomplish a major project have a strong desire to do so. Any significant change begins with a desire for a result or outcome. They have a vision of what they want to accomplish.

Intend: The next step in the sequence is to translate a strong desire into a compelling intention—the will to do something to accomplish the desire. An intention enhances the strength, the pull, of the desire by transforming it into a possibility.

Want: When desire is coupled with intention, a strong sense of wanting follows. Now the outcome is more than just wishful thinking. The individual wants to fulfill the intention.

Can: When people want to achieve a result, they will move forward only if they believe they have the capacity to do so—a can-do attitude.

Allow: A belief in one's capability must be followed by internal permission. People must give themselves permission to change. They must give themselves permission to undertake the project and reach success. This step is crucial in that those who approach a project with equivocation or doubt or incongruence will not give themselves permission to succeed. Instead, they will, perhaps unknowingly, sabotage their own success.

Decide/choose: People who give themselves permission to succeed then make choices that promote progress and support the outcome.

Put in motion: Making decisions and choices is not sufficient to accomplish a result. Successful individuals implement their decisions and choices with action.

Sustain the effort: Putting a plan into motion does not bring success unless one also sustains the effort sufficiently to reach the outcome.

Complete: People succeed when they have put forth sustained action sufficient to complete the project. In the case of weight reduction, the project is accomplished when the individual reaches his or her target weight. Now the project shifts from weight reduction to weight maintenance. In this manner, the results are preserved.

If your client is not making progress and seems stuck, then you want to determine where the sticking point lies. You could ask questions addressing each link in the chain. Here are examples:

Desire: At this point, do you still desire a healthy weight?

Intend: What do you intend to do in order to accomplish that result?

Want: What do you want as your plan? What steps and stipulations are in the plan?

Can: Do you believe you can carry out the plan effectively, even though you may have to make adjustments to the plan along the way?

Allow: Do you have any concerns, hesitations, or conflicts that might deter you from the plan? Do you congruently give yourself permission to carry out the plan? Do you congruently give yourself permission to have the result?

Decide/choose: Do you now decide to move forward? What additional decisions will you make in order to have your plan lead to success?

Put in motion: What actions will you take? Where, when, how, how long, and how often?

Sustain the effort: What resources will help you sustain the effort sufficiently to get the results you envision?

Complete: How will you know precisely when you have accomplished your result? At that point, given the amount of effort you've put forth to accomplish the result, and how important it is to you, would you be willing then to develop a plan for weight maintenance?

A sticking point usually occurs when the individual encounters an unforeseen conflict, setback, or obstacle. Ultimately, the client always has the option to bow out and resign from the project. You cannot force someone to make a change he or she no longer wants. Ascertain whether the client's response is true resignation or merely discouragement. If the client truly wants to drop the effort at this time, respect the client's decision and go no further, except to offer your services in the future under better circumstances.

The case more often is that the client has run up against some impasse and does not know how to resolve it. Ask, "In spite of this setback/conflict/obstacle, is it still worth it to you to reach your target weight?" If the answer is yes, ask, "Are you willing to find a way to work through this difficulty and resolve it, even if it means making some changes to your plan?" If the answer is again yes, this is the point at which the two of you can explore options and possibilities in order to develop solutions.

German philosopher Friedrich Nietzsche once said, "He who has a strong enough why can bear with almost any how." A compelling, realistic, well-formed outcome is often powerful enough to get one through almost any impasse. So one step is to help the client find a compelling value associated with the target weight—a value that overrides discouragement.

Here's one method to enhance the client's desire and create a strong intention. Some people who are overweight have trouble imagining what it's really like to have a healthy weight. They maintain an image of themselves as fat, even while endeavoring to lose weight. Without a clear vision of what is possible, they are easily discouraged and distracted from obtaining the outcome. Have the client envision a future self at the desired weight and size. Employ guided imagery, instructing the client to step into the image and imagine living it fully. Here is a sample script:

> Step into the image and be there now. You've continued with your plan, despite setbacks, and you are thrilled with your success! Now you are living your life in a healthier body. No more lugging around all that fat! You walk differently now. You think differently now. You feel different now. Imagine the size and style of clothing you are wearing now. See yourself in a full-length mirror and imagine the pleasure of looking fit, healthy, and confident. You have more energy. It's easy to bend over to tie your shoelace. It's easy to get in and out of a car. Imagine walking down a street and catching a glimpse of yourself reflected in a shop window, and you have to look twice, just to make sure it's you, because you look so much more attractive. A smile comes to your face and a lightness to your step. Imagine that you run into a friend who hasn't seen you for a while. You can see the surprise on her face as she says "Wow! You look fantastic!" You enjoy a glow of satisfaction over what you have accomplished and you say, "It was tough, but it's worth it, to look and feel this good!" It's so liberating, you feel empowered to do

things you were afraid to do before, when you were heavy. Now you have the confidence and courage to consider new possibilities.

Now bring the client's attention back to the present and ask, "What else will having the weight you desire do for you—something even more significant than all these benefits?" Follow the outcome chain described in chapter 6. For each response the client gives, keep asking, "And what does having/doing that do for you that is even more meaningful?" This line of questioning elicits a hierarchy of values that supports the outcome. Keep asking the question until the client identifies a value that is sufficient to motivate him or her to work through the impasse. When the value is identified, make a statement that succinctly links the value to the outcome in a powerful way.

For instance, let's say the identified value is "responsibility." Your reflective remarks would be similar to these:

> I hear you saying that your sense of responsibility is a driving force in all the meaningful things you do, is that correct? Does that mean, then, that to accomplish anything less than what you have set out to do would constitute an act of irresponsibility on your part? Do you agree that your progress in accomplishing the weight you choose is deeply tied to your sense of responsibility? How much more motivated do you feel now that you realize this sense of responsibility? May I ask you to take responsibility for figuring out how to resolve this difficulty and move forward? Are you willing to explore some solutions?

Once the client agrees to explore solutions, ask questions that prompt creative thinking about getting past the block:

> What would make it possible for you to resolve this difficulty and continue making progress? What else? What else? What is the most viable option at this point? What is your plan to implement that option? What is the next step to take? How will you carry out that step? When will you do it?

By the way, if the client feels stuck but cannot identify the source of the impasse, then the block is probably due not to some external circumstance in the client's life, but more likely to some unconscious inhibition. Go to the Six-Step Reframe, described in chapter 7. Use this process to work with "the part of you that has kept you stuck and not making headway." The positive intention might reveal the underlying cause of the impasse.

Resolving the impasse often requires changing the plan or changing the parameters of the project. You might also find that moving through the impasse requires a separate itinerary of change, nested in the structure of the larger process. Cycling through the links in the chain again (this time to resolve the impasse) helps the client break the larger change process into smaller and smaller chunks until the "next step" is doable.

Reframing Failure

Failure can constitute a formidable obstacle to progress in any significant endeavor. In weight reduction, failure occurs when people eat too much or neglect exercise sufficiently that they prevent weight reduction, or worse, they gain weight. Such a failure often stops people in their tracks—unless they have a strategy to keep going. Discouragement, resignation, and giving up may ensue. Failure may create an "I can't" belief. There is a strategy for reframing failure into an element of the process for achieving success.

In their outstanding book *The NLP Coach*, coaching consultants, trainers, and NLP experts Ian McDermott and Wendy Jago (2001), discuss the structure of failure and of success in any endeavor. They write, "Failure doesn't just happen—it has structure and sequence. ... Failures are ... the results of interactions in a system. ... NLP takes a systemic view of things. This means looking at the different elements in a situation as parts of a system that function for good or ill. Once you understand how the system is working—for or against you—you have a means of structuring things differently in the future" (p. 87).

McDermott and Jago posit a relationship between people's actions and the results they get. Both success and failure leave a trail of clues as to what went right and what went wrong. People who succeed in accomplishing their outcomes have a distinctive response to failure: They examine it with curiosity to retrieve useful information that they can use in modifying their plan and making different choices. They define failure as an unexpected "detour" in the journey toward the desired outcome. The detour may make the journey longer and more arduous, but eventually they get back on track and keep going.

Conversely, other people may regard failure as a reason to dispense with the project altogether. They may perceive failure as an indication of personal inadequacy, inability, or incompetence. They may take failure as confirmation that they are unworthy of the outcome or that the process is too difficult, perhaps impossible. They may conclude that the odds are stacked against their success. Worse yet, some people, once they fail, keep repeating the behaviors that led to failure in the first place, each time hoping for (but not getting) a different result. Some people may decide that the outcome isn't worth the effort or may deny how much they really desire the outcome, because it seems farther and farther out of reach. These responses to failure cause people to give in to defeat and give up.

McDermott and Jago write,

> You will undoubtedly learn something from every "failure." The only question is, is it a good learning? Failures can be belief-forming because we draw conclusions from them, and these conclusions guide our future feelings and actions. If

failure leads to self-blame or a sense of worthlessness, it can restrict ambition, bring on depression, and perhaps further damage our self-image. This can lead to anger and bitterness, cynicism, or a deviant and revengeful attitude to others, authority, or even society in general (p. 94).

A crucial element in the structure of success in any endeavor is to regard "failure" (lack of success) as a source of feedback. The concept is also a basic presupposition in the practice of NLP. You can model curiosity to coach your client beyond failure. Curiosity regards the failure event as an opportunity to acquire more information about how to succeed. Curiosity expresses itself as questions like these:

- How did you get this result?
- Where did the mistakes occur?
- What were the circumstances?
- What were you thinking about that led you to that choice?
- What did you do that was useful?
- What did you do that was not useful?
- What other factors were involved—people, timing, location?
- What were you most aware of when things went wrong?
- Was there anything you could have been more aware of?

Notice that the questions focus on behaviors, thoughts, and feelings. This is important because some people have a tendency to think of failure as a definition of self—a matter of identity. Instead of saying, "I failed at staying on the plan," they say, "I am a failure." Additionally, ask for specificity. Don't accept, "I just messed up." Don't allow the client to generalize or go global with the information, as in, "Well, I can't do anything right, and I always eat too much." (Hint from your NLP training: This is where the Meta-Model comes in handy. See chapter 17 for more information.)

When you have a description of what went wrong, look for the crucial details that made the difference between success and failure. Try out various scenarios: "If this one element had been different, would the result have been the same?" Richard Bandler and John Grinder developed NLP by asking the essential question, "What is the difference that makes the difference?" With specific information about what contributed to the "failure," you and your client can reconstruct the strategy or chain of events that led to the failure and determine what corrections are needed. Now go to these types of questions about the possible solutions for the future:

- What are other possible ways to handle this kind of situation?
- What do you want to do differently from now on, in those circumstances?
- How will you make this change?
- How will your thinking, emotions, and actions be different?

- What additional resources or information would be of benefit?
- What will help you remember to do things in this new way?
- How do you think you'll feel with a different result?
- Will this change be sufficient to get you back on track?
- Is there anything else you'd want to do?
- Is this new way of handling things suitable to you?
- Are you ready to recommit to having the weight you desire, and to add this new behavioral strategy to your repertoire?

Accountability

Have you ever had the experience of your client agreeing to carry out an assigned task or engage in a new behavior, and then returning for the next session without having completed the assignment? When you ask if he or she followed through on the new behavior or the assignment, here are some of the answers you might get:

"I was supposed to do that? I don't remember it!"

"Gee, I don't know. I guess I just forgot."

"Well, I got busy with other things, and I didn't think it was that important, and I ran out of time."

Don't blame your client. A basic presupposition of NLP is that the response you get is a result of the way you communicate. The responsibility for making oneself understood lies with the person doing the communicating. Our clients come to therapy and counseling because they don't know how to manage aspects of their lives. Often, they don't know how to consistently manage their thoughts, emotions, behaviors, time, relationships, and resources in such a way as to achieve some specific outcome. That's why they have come to you in the first place! Lack of follow-through is an all-too-common human trait.

Your client planned to succeed, but got bogged down in the process. Unanticipated problems and obstacles have reared their ugly heads. Together, the two of you have decided on some solutions to the problems and modified the plan. The client has agreed to take action, but doesn't keep the agreement. What do you do now?

Take another cue from coaching and ask for accountability. According to Laura Whitworth, Henry Kimsey-House, and Phil Sandahl, authors of *Co-Active Coaching* (1998, p. 253), accountability means "having our clients account for what they said they were going to do." For the client, accountability becomes a motivating factor, because it involves another person in the process of achieving an outcome. There is someone monitoring progress. The simple act of giv-ing one's word to someone raises the stakes and increases motivation. It creates focus and discipline. Accountability rests on four questions:

1. What are you going to do?
2. What are the specific steps you will take?
3. By when will you do this?
4. How will I know you have done it?

Then ask, "Do I have your permission to hold you accountable for this?" If the answer is yes, then ask, "Do you then agree that I can hold you to account for your vision and commitment to your intended action?" If your client has a his-tory of laxity in maintaining agreements, get the agreement in writing and give one copy to the client and keep one for yourself. Explore what will be different this time when the client keeps the agreement instead of shrugging it off.

Accountability is not about nagging, reminding, blaming, judging, scolding, or punishing. It is eliciting feedback. It is asking for information. "What result did you get? What worked? What didn't work? What could you do differently next time?" With these types of questions, you and the client might identify addi-tional sticking points or misunderstandings. You and the client could brain-storm possible solutions, modify the plan, choose another strategy, or devise an educational between-session assignment.

Whitworth, Kimsey-House, and Sandahl (1998) write, "Co-active coaches are not attached to the result clients achieve. … Coaches want their clients to excel, of course … but the results belong to the client. … As coaches, we hold clients accountable—not to see them perform or how well they perform, but to empower the change they want to make. Accountability can provide the means for change and creates a great opportunity to acknowledge how they succeed" (p. 82). Accountability sets the expectation that clients will do what they say they will do. It means you *notice* whether or not they follow through on agree-ments and commitments.

On occasion, you might sense that the client is testing the boundaries of accountability to determine whether you really will hold to the agreement. If the client doesn't fully carry out the agreement, the accountability issue itself becomes "grist for the mill." You say, "I'm aware that you didn't do what you said you'd do. How do you want to handle being accountable in this relation-ship? What matters to you in keeping this agreement? What structures and resources, rewards and consequences would you want in place that would be sufficient to motivate you to keep the agreement?" These questions put the ball squarely in the client's court to take action and assume responsibility for his or her agenda.

Tips for Working with Clients Who Don't Exercise

Getting regular, consistent exercise is often a sticking point for people who are overweight. Most people I've met who don't exercise give one of two reasons: (a) they have trouble finding time to exercise, or (b) they don't enjoy it. They usually don't enjoy it because they find it difficult, painful, and fatiguing. The next four paragraphs describe how to handle the exercise issue.

If your client has trouble scheduling time to exercise, then explore time-management issues. Planning to exercise "whenever I have spare time" will not work. Defining exercise as a "spare time" activity makes exercise an optional activity in competition with other "spare time" tasks, such as cleaning out the closets. The only way to make exercise a regular activity is to schedule it as an appointment. That's why some people join an exercise class—because the class schedule gives a structure to "time for exercise." If the client faces other priorities that conflict with exercise time, help the client find ways to negotiate the conflict. Suppose your client says, "I want to go to the gym, but I don't want to leave my child at home alone." Then talk about having a friend over to stay with the child or finding a gym with a day-care center or devising ways to exercise at home and include the child in the activity. Explore the options and find a solution.

If the client does not enjoy exercise, suggest finding a way of exercising that is enjoyable. Exercising may be more enjoyable with companions, when set to music, or when done out of doors or while watching television. One client may hate walking in place but enjoy a ballroom dancing class. Another approach is to point out that we often do things we don't enjoy because, having done those things, we get immense satisfaction from the fact that we have undergone some momentary discomfort in order to accomplish a highly valued result. You may hate flossing your teeth, but you do it because it prevents gum infections. Perhaps you forgo a few luxury purchases in order to save money for a comfortable retirement.

Use the guidelines from the report in appendix J: "The Benefits of Exercise" to help the client choose an exercise plan that is doable. One problem may be that the client has exaggerated expectations. Perhaps, for example, a sedentary client expects to run a mile each day. Encourage the client just to walk a few blocks (or whatever distance is comfortable) for the first week and then add short distances as strength allows.

For clients who are experiencing health problems that curtail or limit their exercise activities, advise them to check with their physician or a physical trainer as to what kinds of exercise might be suitable. For example, a client with bad knees may not be able to walk distances but could still do some upper body activity while sitting down or could swim or do water exercises, since the water supports the body's weight, greatly reducing joint stress.

When All Else Fails, Make a Referral

Keep in mind that weight control is a problem of a physical as well as a cognitive-behavioral nature. When your client is following the plan for nutrition and exercise precisely and still is not reducing weight, it's time to refer. Make a referral to a bariatric physician in your area for a full-scale medical examination. If your client doesn't want to go to a bariatric physician or is already under the care of a competent physician, then refer to a nutritionist for a re-evaluation of the nutrition plan.

Joe (not his real name) had completed the fourth session in the WHY Program when he left a message on my answering machine that he couldn't keep the appointment for the fifth session. I phoned him back and asked him why he cancelled. He said he was keeping his calorie count low and walking a mile every day, but still was not losing weight. I asked questions about sleep, exercise, and stress in his life. Everything was going okay on those fronts. I gave him the name of a nutritionist who could go over his food plan with him to find anything that might be slowing his weight reduction. A few weeks later Joe called me and made the appointment. He had reduced his weight by ten pounds. He said the nutritionist had identified some flaws in his calorie counting and his food plan, which he easily corrected.

Chapter 16

More NLP Patterns for Changing Compulsive Eating

"I was doing fine until Friday night, when I went out with friends and just pigged out."

"Well, last week I wanted something sweet, so I thought I would have just a little bit of ice cream. But once I got started, I couldn't stop. I ate the whole half gallon!"

How often have you heard something like this? People who are overweight cannot give up food entirely the way a smoker can give up cigarettes or an alcoholic, alcohol. They have to deal with food every day—it's always there, and they can't live without it! People who are overweight struggle with the compulsion to eat. Compulsive eating shows up in two ways: (a) overeating all types of food and eating when not hungry, or (b) binge eating a particular type of food, usually sweets or starches—which are highly processed foods. If a client returns again and again to compulsive eating, I recommend that you schedule an extra session in the program to help the client with the problem. You can use any of the NLP patterns in this chapter for that purpose.

Before addressing the problem of overeating or binging, understand that although compulsive eating can be a form of self-soothing, it may also be a symptom of depression, fatigue, an imbalance in blood sugars, or chemical imbalances in the brain, such as reduced serotonin. Neuropsychiatrist Daniel Amen (Amen and Routh 2004) has published several books on the interactions between brain chemistry and lifestyle. He writes that intractable depression, compulsions, and anxiety are sometimes the outward indications of brain-activity dysfunctions caused by factors such as genetics, exposure to toxic substances, adverse drug interactions, drug abuse, trauma, high fevers, head injury, or a poor diet—even though some of these risk factors may have occurred much earlier in one's life. If you suspect your client's compulsive eating may be associated with a brain-activity dysfunction, you may decide to recommend a complete neurological examination. You might also want to share with your client the brain-health recommendations in appendix K (also presented in a report on the *Client Workbook* CD).

To treat compulsive overeating or binge eating with any of the following NLP patterns, begin by getting the client's congruent desire to change the behavior. In the case of overeating, the outcome will most likely be to eat less and to eat only when hungry. In the case of binging, the outcome will be to feel less attracted to the problem food and to eat less of it or none at all. Below are eight NLP patterns for compulsive eating:

1. Pattern interruption
2. Anchoring a new response
3. Mapping across submodalities
4. Eye movements
5. Meta-No and Meta-Yes
7. Swish pattern
8. NLP Slender Eating Strategy.

A word of caution: When applying any of these patterns, be alert for ecological considerations and be ready to address them if they arise. If the client reports distress during any process, stop, explore the distress, and modify the pattern accordingly or choose another pattern.

Pattern Interruption

In the book *Ordeal Therapy* (1984), Jay Haley documented several cases in which Dr. Milton H. Erickson helped his patients create change by giving them strange or unusual assignments to perform outside of therapy sessions. In these assignments, clients were instructed to alter their normal patterns around their problem behaviors in such a way that they learned something new and extinguished the problem. One of Erickson's most frequent assignments, when he was living in Phoenix, Arizona, was telling a client or student to climb nearby Piestewa Peak (formerly called Squaw Peak) and return with a new perspective on the presented problem.

In writing about the basic concepts of ordeal therapy, Overdurf and Silverthorn (1995) state that the purpose of each assignment is to interrupt the client's existing pattern from a structural point of view:

> The key to designing ordeals is based upon Meta-Programs, values, and strategies. The fundamental question ... is, "What have you tried to do (to solve this problem) that hasn't worked?" Exhaust all possible answers and write them down. Look at the sequence of events. What has to follow what? ... Set aside the notion of cause and effect and think instead in terms of loops. ... The result is that the point of intervention will not be directed at the source of the problem (the cause) but rather how the client attempts to solve the problem. ... The intervention itself needs to be a behavior ... that presupposes either the outcome for the therapy or some other positive result which is different from the problem. (p. 30).

If you like working in this way, follow these guidelines:

1. Tell the client you will give an assignment that will change the way he or she thinks and feels about binging or overeating. Persuade the client to commit to carry out the assignment consistently and to be held accountable for doing so.

2. Elicit the client's pattern of overeating or binging. Listen for visual or auditory triggers, such as seeing a plate of pastries at the office or being at a party and seeing food on the buffet table. Maybe the trigger is the client's spouse saying, "Let's go out for ice cream." Ask for the client's internal dialogue and representations, mind-body state, and decision points.

3. Design an assignment that alters the client's normal pattern of compulsive eating. When you give the assignment, obtain the client's commitment to carry out this task, with the clear understanding it is neither hurtful nor a punishment but an educational experience, designed to help the client relinquish a behavior. Use the accountability strategy in chapter 15 to encourage the client to complete the assignment.

Here are a few examples of assignments you might give:

•   Each time the client binges on any given food, he or she must, within 24 hours, purchase twice that amount of the same food and throw it away immediately. For each additional instance of binging, the client must double the amount of food purchased and thrown away. Each time the client binges, he or she must contact you within 24 hours to report having carried out the assignment.

•   The client keeps a food journal and makes an entry each time he or she eats. Each type of food must be measured and recorded. The client must purchase a calorie counter (these small hand-held computer/calculator devices can be purchased over the Internet) and record the number of calories for each type of food eaten.

•   The client can eat as much food as he or she wants but must eat only when sitting at the kitchen table (or at his or her desk at work), alone, with no distractions—no newspapers, no television or radio, no computer, no books or mail to read. The client must eat slowly and concentrate on nothing but the act of eating.

•   Clients agree to designate one day each week when they totally ignore the nutrition plan and eat whatever they please, as long as they stick with the plan the other six days of the week. They must plan in advance which day will be the day off the plan. In this way, improper eating is no longer an automatic, unplanned activity, but is arranged in advance. Remind clients that reaching their desired weight is about persistence, not perfection. If the client is eating properly six days a week, he or she will still reduce excess pounds.

Anchoring a New Response

Anchoring is described in detail in chapter 9. Anchoring helps someone change a mind-body state in response to a specific stimulus. Here is an anchoring method to help a client feel no attraction at all to a problem food. Before you begin, ascertain that the client wants to feel no attraction at all to this type of food. This pattern is useful for people who have allergic or uncomfortable reactions to specific foods or beverages or have been advised by their physician to avoid specific foods or beverages.

1. Ask the client to identify some behavior he or she would never do—wouldn't even consider. This behavior should be something against which the client has strong inhibitions and prohibitions, such as cruelty to animals, stealing, or immoral or indecent behavior.

2. When the client expresses something to the effect of "I would never do that!" anchor that response.

3. Ask the client to remember a time of binging on a problem food. Identify the specific external stimulus that prompted binging. Bring the client back to the present moment.

4. Have the client revisit the binging episode. When the client encounters the remembered external stimulus, apply the anchor (that is, the response identified in step 1) *for a different reaction to that food.* Immediately give a new meaning to binging: *"Now you realize it's not a question of whether or not you want ice cream; it's a question of whether you choose discomfort or satisfaction with your decision."* Bring the client's attention back to the present.

5. Have the client rehearse future instances of seeing or thinking about or being reminded of the binge food and feeling repulsed by it or indifferent to it and saying to himself or herself "I would never eat that!"

Mapping across Submodalities

Submodality work (Hall and Bodenhamer [1999a] refer to it as Meta-Detailing) changes the way the client visually represents a problematic type of food, so that the food seems less appealing. In this method, you elicit visual details about the client's image of a disliked food. Then you "map across," applying the same visual details to an image of a problem food—such as sweets, starches, or fatty foods. The following example uses location as a visual submodality. (Location is usually a "driver" detail that exerts significant influence when it is altered.) If the change in location does not yield results, or if both locations are the same, conduct the process with other or additional visual features, such as brightness, color, and size of the image.

1. Ask the client to picture a food or type of food he or she finds distasteful; something he or she would almost never eat. Observe where the client fixes his or her gaze in the visual field. In submodality approaches, this spot is the visual "location." The visual location exists in three dimensions—up-down, right-left, and near-far.

2. Ask the client to picture the problem food or binge food. Again, observe its visual location. Ask the client to rate the attraction to the binge food on a scale from 1 to 10.

3. Tell the client to maintain the image of the binge food and move that image to a new location in the visual field—the location for the disliked food. Calibrate the response. Again, get a 1-to-10 rating for the attraction to it. The rating should be lower this time. If the rating has not changed, or is not low enough (say, a 1 or 2), move the image farther away or to different locations in the visual field, until the rating goes down. You can also instruct the client to change other elements of the image, making it blurry, smaller, washed out, gray, or dim. Sometimes, when one visual element changes, others will change automatically. These changes often diminish the potency of an image, and thus, the attraction of the imaged food.

4. Once you have an image with a low rating, have the client quickly move the image back and forth several times, from the old location to the new location (in NLP this called a "swish"). End with the image in the new location, with any other attendant changes, and tell the client to "make the image stay that way." You can invoke a metaphor such as gluing the new image in place.

5. Have the client rehearse future instances of seeing or thinking about or being reminded of the binge food, calling up the new image, and feeling dislike for or indifference to the binge food.

Eye Movements

Some years ago I attended a workshop by Dr. Connirae Andreas on eye movement integration (EMI). This method is commonly used to neutralize the emotional effects of traumatic events. Dr. Danie Beaulieu has since written *Eye Movement Integration Therapy* (2003) on the topic, and I recommend reading her book for a fuller understanding and appreciation of the method. In a few cases I have used a modified version of EMI for clients who binge, and it seems to work well. Although I cannot state that EMI has efficacy for binge eating based on these few cases, I invite you to experiment with the method to discover whether it works for your clients.

1. Have the client visualize a square or television screen or computer screen in the center of his or her field of vision. Inside the square, have the client visualize the binge food in the way that is most attractive and appealing.

2. Have the client rate his or her level of attraction to the image from 1 to 10. Ask the client to verbalize a "cognition": an immediate thought about the food. The answer might range from attraction, for example, "That looks delicious," to ambivalence, for example, "I wish I didn't like it so much." The client then visualizes the cognition under the image of the problem food, like a caption under a news photo.

3. Tell the client to watch your fingertip as you move it horizontally across the image. Your range of movement should be such that the client moves his or her eyes all the way from one side to another. Make eight to ten sweeps at a pace that is comfortable for you and the client. Stop. Lower your hand and ask the client for a new rating. Ask whether the cognition has changed, and if so, ask the client to state the new cognition. This new cognition goes under the image again, as a caption replacing the previous cognition.

4. Return to the image. Repeat step 3 numerous times, exploring the effect of finger movements in various directions: vertically, diagonally, clockwise, counterclockwise, and figure eights. For each direction of movement, repeat the sweep eight to ten times, then stop, obtain a new rating, and ask about changes in the cognition. In cases where this method has worked, I've heard clients say something to the effect of, "I don't know ... it just doesn't look tasty anymore."

5. Repeat whichever movements yield favorable results. Continue the process until the client's attraction to the binge food reaches a low rating and the cognition is consistent with that low rating.

6. At this point, I ask the client to fixate on the image one more time, while I use hypnotic language patterns to repeat and reinforce the new cognition, to suggest that the food has lost its appeal, that there are other ways to find comfort and enjoyment, and that this change is long lasting. I suggest that when the client encounters this food in the future, the food will have no

meaning, no appeal. It will be "just another type of food" and the client will feel indifferent toward it.

7.   Then I ask the client to make the old image disappear and replace it with an image of herself or himself, healthy and trim, at the desired weight, eating nutritious foods, exercising, and feeling much more confident.

Meta-No and Meta-Yes

Hall and Bodenhamer have written extensively about the use of "Meta-No and Meta-Yes" and have demonstrated the method in their Meta-States and Frame Games books, workshops, and seminars (Hall 2001; Hall and Bodenhamer 2001a). Here I present the method in brief as applied to problem foods or to eating when one is not hungry:

1.   Begin by conditioning a Meta-No. Have the client stand up and reenact various scenarios in which he or she has voiced a very firm and powerful NO!, not to food, but to any stimulus or event where he or she has responded with a definitive NO! Encourage the client to really get into the action, with postures, gestures, and tone of voice and to appreciate fully the ability to say NO! forcefully. The No! should be expressed in various forms, such as an assertive NO!; a gentle, compassionate no, an angry NO WAY!; etc.

2.   Tell the client to visualize the problem food (or better still, have the food on hand), and practice saying various forms of NO! to the problem food. Build the response slowly, by offering the client the food, imploring the client to try it, talking about how delicious it is, and so on. The client continues to voice the various forms of NO!

3.   Praise and support the client for steadfastly saying NO! Explore together how the NO! could be even more powerful and effective. Have the client practice even more powerful ways of saying NO! to problem foods, until he or she has a strong internal NO!

4.   Coach the client to act out and rehearse socially acceptable responses in various contexts (parties, picnics, and so on) where he or she now can easily refuse or avoid the problem food.

5.   Now switch to Meta-Yes! Have the client imagine various scenarios of activities he or she really enjoys. These activities might be having sex, listening to favorite music, taking a hot shower or bubble bath, or a favorite sport. For each activity, have the client demonstrate saying an affirmative,

congruent YES! Again, elicit various form of YES! and encourage him or her to really get into the action.

6. Tell the client to visualize healthful alternative foods (such as salads, vegetables, or fruits) and practice saying a strong, powerful YES! to these foods.

Other potentially useful Frame Games and Meta-States methods from Bodenhamer (2004) and Hall (2000) for overeating or binge eating are described below. I suggest you read Bodenhamer for a fuller explanation of these patterns.

Drop down and through: This method uses the presupposition that emotions can exist in layers, with each layer taking the individual to a different feeling about the previous layer. Take the individual "down and through" a troubling emotion as a way to incorporate the emotion within the context of a broader and more extensive resource. For example, if the client's emotion is boredom say, "Drop down through the bored feeling to discover what lies beneath the boredom. What do you experience now?" Keep dropping down through layers of emotion until the client reaches a resourceful state—usually a core state of spirituality, identity, belief, or value. Now anchor this core state and apply the anchor to the preceding states, in reverse order. This process transforms and neutralizes the troubling emotions that originally led to some maladaptive behavior, such as binge eating.

Mind-to-muscle: Help the client articulate a highly valued belief that supports the outcome. Use anchors to chain the highly valued belief into a decision, then into an anticipatory experience, based on the decision, then into a plan, then into an action, and then to a commitment to the action with motivation and excitement.

Emotional intensity installation: Install a highly charged, positive emotional state around a specific and desired frame of thinking and behaving about food and eating. Have the client mentally rehearse having this response in the future in specific contexts where binging was the previous response.

Miracle installation: Based on de Shazer's "Miracle Question" (1988), this pattern prompts the listener to imagine going to bed at night, and during the night a miracle occurs, and he or she wakes up in the morning, having fully achieved the outcome and all its attendant consequences and rewards. Gather detailed information from the client about all the changes that would occur. Then use hypnosis and guided imagery to help the client imagine having all the changes, one by one: enjoying the rewards, coping with the consequences, and maintaining new behaviors, thoughts, beliefs, and attitudes. End the session by encouraging the client to act, in the real world, as if the miracle has already taken place.

Genius frame: Teach the client to access highly committed and passionate states and to appoint an "executive" ego state to decide the contexts in which each these states are useful and will be applied when making choices about food.

Swish Pattern

Use the swish pattern for clients who overeat or binge to cope with uncomfortable emotions. It was developed by Richard Bandler (1985). In the swish pattern, the client visualizes a self-image that is sufficiently resourceful (a) to avoid binging or overeating, and (b) to manage stressful emotions in healthy ways. The swish pattern is a pattern interruption that installs a new coping strategy. There are many variations on the swish pattern. Here is one.

1. Have the client access a memory of a recent binging episode. Identify the problem context. Elicit the client's visual external trigger for binging and his or her internal state just before deciding to binge. Stop the memory at that point.

2. Bring the client's attention back to the present and instruct him or her to create a dissociated image of a more resourceful self (context-free). This imagined self is capable of handling any similar situation competently, without turning to food as a pacifier. Ask the client to describe the traits this version of self possesses, such as confidence, power, and assertiveness. Encourage the client to alter the submodalities until the image is attractive, rich, and compelling and evokes positive feelings.

3. Shrink the resourceful-state image developed in step 2 down to a small icon that the client maintains in the lower right-hand corner of his or her visual field. Some NLP practitioners use the analogy of a computer file that can be reduced to a small folder that remains on the computer desktop, ready to be reopened in an instant.

4. This step takes place very quickly, in mere seconds. Again, have the client access the problem context in step 1. This time, however, at the trigger point, have the client mentally open the file of the resourceful image and visualize a self who is perfectly competent to handle the situation resourcefully. The image of a resourceful self quickly gets bigger and brighter until it blots out the image of the remembered problem context, which in turn, gets dim and shrinks: "See the image of a competent, powerful you, and take in all these resources and qualities, as you absorb and become this

resourceful image of yourself, knowing you can handle the situation effectively." Some NLP practitioners add a swooshing "sound effect" to signify the transposition of the two images. Suggest to the client that while viewing the resourceful self, he or she will activate those resources within.

5. Clear the client's visual field. Repeat step 4 five times, clearing the visual field after each repetition. Encourage the client to perform the step very quickly, with progressively less instruction each time, "so that you can do this on your own."

6. Test. Have the client reassociate to the original memory (as in step 1) and "try, in vain, to get back the old feelings and find you cannot access them."

7. Guide the client in future rehearsal of possible challenging situations where he or she will use the swish strategy—focusing on an image of a resourceful self, activating the resources, and applying those resources in the challenging situation.

Naturally Slender Eating Strategy

The Naturally Slender Eating Strategy was developed by Steve and Connirae Andreas and described in their book *Heart of the Mind* (1989). A variation of the strategy that I have used with many clients appears on the *Client Workbook* CD (as the assignment for session 6) and in appendix I for quick reference. You can also teach this strategy to your client in a face-to-face session.

Chapter 17

Advanced NLP Language Patterns

Sadly, the people most afflicted by obesity are also the least likely to want to exercise or eat intelligently. In conversations, phone calls, and face-to-face sessions with clients who are overweight, you'll want to maintain an ample repertoire of advanced language patterns to redirect negative thinking and continue to persuade, influence, and motivate them to maintain their commitment to a healthy lifestyle. This chapter offers examples and advice on using advanced NLP language patterns to lend additional support to client outcomes. The language pattern domains are the Meta-Model, Sleight of Mouth Patterns, Meta-Programs, metaphors and analogies, languaging the past and present (verb tense), and solution-oriented questions.

Meta-Model

The purpose of the Meta-Model is to bring precision to the client's thinking and communicating. For the practitioner, it is a method of therapeutic inquiry about the client's conversation designed to elicit specificity, clear up confusion, and challenge unclear communication (and thinking) by uncovering deletions, distortions, generalizations, and presuppositions. Many authors in the field of NLP have written extensively about the Meta-Model, and I will not go into background or detail here, except to remind you that the Meta-Model can be used to address, clarify, and challenge many of the common thinking patterns of clients who are overweight. Consider the following examples where Meta-Model responses follow a client's assertion.

Client: *Food is my source of comfort*

Simple Deletions
- How much food do you have to eat in order to feel comfortable?
- What is it exactly about food that you associate with comfort?
- How long does the comfort from food last?

Distortions
Nominalization: How exactly do you comfort yourself with food?

Complex equivalent: What will happen when you begin to think of food as a source of nutrition instead of comfort?

Cause-and-effect: What do you tell yourself that makes you think food is comforting?

Generalizations
Static words: Which specific food or foods are your source of comfort?

Multi-ordinal words: What definition of comfort are you using?

Universal quantifiers: Is food your only source of comfort? Do you have no other options? Do you always comfort yourself with food?

Presuppositions
• Do you presuppose food has some magical ability to comfort you?
• What if comfort is only the result of associations you've learned in the past?
• Are you saying you have no other way to get comfort?
• What does comfort have to do with overeating and gaining weight?

Client: *I just can't seem to stick to my food/exercise plan*

Simple Deletions
• When, exactly, are you not sticking to your plan?
• What is your plan, specifically?
• What prevents you from sticking to your plan?
• In what way do you keep yourself from sticking to your plan?

Distortions
Unspecified verbs: How would you know if you were sticking to your plan?

Nominalization: How exactly do you plan to eat and exercise?

Modal operators: Is it possible for you to stick to your plan?

Generalizations
Multi-ordinal words: What specific parts of the plan are you not sticking to?

Universal quantifiers: You haven't stuck to it at all?

Presuppositions
• Are you assuming you have to stick with the plan perfectly for it to work?
• Is there a way to modify your plan so that you could stick with it?

Client: *I eat whether or not I feel hungry*

Deletions
- If you eat whether or not you feel hungry, when do you eat and how much?
- What do you eat exactly?
- If you don't feel hungry when you eat, what do you feel instead?

Distortions
Unspecified adjectives: How do you know whether or not you feel hungry?

Modal operators: Do you *have* to eat, whether or not you are hungry?

Delusional verbal splits: Are you saying that eating has nothing to do with your bodily sensations?

Cause-and-effect: Are you saying you eat food just because it's there? Does that mean the mere presence of food causes you to eat?

Generalizations
Universal quantifiers: Do you always eat, never stopping and without exception?

Presuppositions
- You have no choice, no decision in the matter?
- What if you decide to eat only when you feel hungry?
- What if you allow yourself to get hungry so that you can make the distinction?
- What is the purpose of eating, if not in response to hunger?

By challenging and questioning the client's limiting assertions through the Meta-Model, it is possible to reveal an inner map of limitations that have kept the person locked into overeating and obesity. This map can be a starting point for therapeutic discussions and interventions.

Sleight of Mouth Patterns

Sleight of Mouth Patterns are useful conversational ploys to expand people's thinking and send their thoughts in new directions. When delivering these patterns, be careful that your tone of voice does not sound judgmental, sarcastic, or critical. Here are some examples for a client who says "I just don't feel like exercising."

Redefine: If you don't feel like it, maybe that means you haven't yet found a way to exercise that works for you. Let's talk about that.

Consequence: I guess some days it's a matter of figuring out which is worse, feeling lousy while exercising or feeling lousy every time you look in the mirror!

Intention: What does not exercising do for you?

Chunk down: What specific aspect of exercising do you not feel like doing?

Chunk up: Have you ever thought about what your life would be like if you always opted out, just because you didn't feel like doing something?

Counterexample: When "you don't feel like it" is probably the best time to examine your priorities and ask yourself whether your exercise plan is really working for you.

Another outcome: Let me propose that the issue is not how you feel on any given day; it's your commitment to being healthy, fulfilling a responsibility to yourself, and having the freedom to move more easily and carry yourself with more confidence. Are you still committed to those outcomes?

Metaphor: That's like a mother saying to her baby, "I don't feel like feeding you or changing your diapers today." (Use an example that matches the client's responsibilities to a spouse, a child, a job, a pet, or a friend.)

Apply the criterion to itself: The secret to getting your target weight is to *not like* the feeling of not feeling like exercising ... and to not like it so much that you actually *do* feel like exercising, because you like the feeling of feeling like exercising.

Hierarchy of criteria: Being a grown-up means realizing that sometimes it's worth doing things we don't like because the rewards are so satisfying, and the consequences of not doing them become intolerable.

Change frame size: How does the discomfort and inconvenience of exercise compare to the benefits of increasing your metabolism, boosting your energy, and getting healthier?

Meta-Frame: When you say you don't feel like exercising, how, then, do you feel about your commitment to reducing your weight?

Model of the world: Some people don't even consider whether or not they feel like it. Exercising is just a given—like earning a living, paying bills, and taking care of one's children.

Reality strategy: Do you have ways to get yourself to do something, even when, at first, you don't feel like doing it?

Obviously, you could apply similar Sleight of Mouth Patterns to excuses about not eating low-fat foods or not making a full commitment to weight reduction. For more information on Sleight of Mouth Patterns, consider reading *Mind Lines: Lines for Changing Minds*, by Hall and Bodenhamer (2001b).

Meta-Programs

In *Think Yourself Slim*, NLP master practitioner Carol Harris (1999) has written that approaches to weight management should take into account personal motivation and performance patterns—also known as Meta-Programs. Her book examines goal setting, behavior, thought patterns, feelings, and beliefs as essential factors in motivation. During conversations with your clients, listen for their Meta-Programs and use those Meta-Programs as leverage points for motivation. When you recognize your clients' primary Meta-Programs, you can choose words and phrases that match well with the ways they motivate themselves. Harris names ten Meta-Program distinctions that have a bearing on how people organize their thoughts and behaviors to change their eating and exercise habits:

Motivational level: finding it difficult versus easy to get going on important tasks

Preference for thinking or taking action: tending to contemplate a task or project before beginning it (reflective), versus jumping in and getting started right away (proactive)

Time orientation: thinking oriented mostly toward the past, present, or future

Primary sensory modality: using a preferred modality for processing and representing information; namely, visual, auditory, kinesthetic, or "internal"

Attitude toward new things: being cautious versus willing to experiment and take risks in undertaking new tasks and projects

Self-reliance (frame of reference): preferring to receive feedback and validation from others (sorting by others) versus acting based on one's own opinion (sorting by self)

Sociability: preferring to work alone versus with other people

Direction of motivation: striving to achieve targets (toward) versus to avoid problems (away from)

Options or procedures: tending to consider options versus following set procedures and rules

Global versus detail: tending to process information at the global level versus at the detail level

The following paragraphs briefly discuss how to work with each type within the ten Meta-Programs. Remember, however, that some people may present a mix of types or fall somewhere in the middle of these traits. There are many more Meta-Programs than the few mentioned here, and all could have some bearing on motivation to manage weight, eat sensibly, exercise, and undertake health-promoting behaviors.

Motivational Level

A client with a high or low motivation level is generally easy to recognize; just ask how he or she typically feels about taking on new projects and challenges.

- Obviously, clients with high motivational levels start a weight reduction program with much enthusiasm and may be excited by the novelty of a new approach or a new beginning.

- Clients with low motivational levels need a great deal of encouragement and support. They benefit from learning how to motivate themselves through using positive self-talk, identifying role models who have successfully reduced their weight, and visualizing their goals and outcomes vividly.

Preference for Thinking or Taking Action

If you aren't sure of the client's tendency, ask, "When you start a new project, do you usually take action right away, or think things over first?"

- When working with reflective clients, recognize and respect their need to "take time to think things over" before taking action. They don't like feeling pushed into action before they are ready. One strategy is to propose a time frame for making a decision. You could say, "Why don't you think about this for a few days, and call me on Friday with your decision and your outline for a plan of action?"

• For people who tend to take action immediately, help them first develop a plan of action outlining the sequence of steps that will lead to the result. Be prepared to help them revise the plan when they run into unforeseen delays, detours, and setbacks.

Time Orientation

What is the client's main time orientation for making major decisions? For people who tend to think mainly in the past, the present, or the future, your task is to help them effectively represent and process all three time zones in a resourceful manner. The book *Time Lining* (Bodenhamer and Hall 1997b) presents many tools and methods for engaging time productively. To effectively undertake any major life change, it is helpful to

• draw upon past successes and lessons learned; access resources from past achievements; and relinquish the negative effects of past failures, disappointments, and trauma.

• decide, in each present moment, what is urgent; what is important and consistent with short-term and long-term outcomes; and what activities constitute the best use of one's time. It's also beneficial to celebrate successes as they occur and cherish precious, meaningful moments that will not happen again.

• see future options, possibilities, and contingencies; plan the steps for accomplishing desired outcomes; and feel motivated by the rewards and greater sense of fulfillment that await.

Primary Sensory Modality

Does the client process information via mainly visual, auditory, kinesthetic, or internal dialogue channels? Listen for the predicates he or she uses and you'll have the answer. Visual predicates are visually oriented words and phrases such as "see," "look," "envision," "show," "appear," "shiny," "dim," "eyeball," "look in the eye," and so on. Auditory predicates resonate with words such as "hear," "say," "tell," "listen," "sounds like," "echo," "chime in," "music to my ears," and so on. Kinesthetic words and phrases refer to body sensations, physical movement, and feelings ("grasp," "get a feel for," "cool off," "warm up to," "yearn for," "get a kick out of," "let go," "hold on," "push the envelope," "get into a comfort zone," and so on). Internal processing refers to figuring things out via internal dialogue ("turning it over in my mind," "thinking it over," "mulling it over," "concentrating on it," "processing it," and so on).

When it comes to motivation, goals and outcomes seem more real, appealing, and doable when all senses are involved, so help your client begin with his or her primary sensory system, followed by the other three. In other words, to accomplish an important goal, it's useful to see oneself doing it; pair the vision with motivating words, phrases, sounds, and music; imagine and anticipate the positive feelings and sensations; and talk to oneself about it.

- Help visual clients focus on the importance of looking attractive and professional to themselves and others. Help them maintain clear, compelling images of the results they want.

- Ask auditory clients, "What would you like to hear that will give you even more motivation?" and "What will your friends say when they see all that weight coming off?" These clients are very careful to articulate their thoughts and ideas clearly. Words are important to auditory clients, so don't substitute your words for theirs. Use their wording instead, to establish rapport and stay in pace with them during the conversation. They might also enjoy exercising or relaxing to appropriate music.

- If your client tends toward the kinesthetic (and many obese people are kinesthetic), put heavy emphasis on the hardships of aching joints, lugging around that heavy burden, and trudging and struggling to get up a staircase; and conversely, the great feelings that accompany weight reduction—feeling confident and energetic, moving around more easily, breathing easily and more comfortably—bending and stretching with much more freedom, agility, and flexibility.

- For clients who process internally, ask, "What do you say to yourself about _____" (weight, nutrition, exercise, plans, outcomes, setbacks and obstacles, and so on). You might help them change that internal dialogue to make it more motivating, positive, future-oriented, congruent, and realistic.

Attitude toward New Things

When it comes to working with you on the WHY Program, does the client ask for proof or prefer to move forward on the basis of personal experience?

- A cautious person wants proven methods for weight control. This type of person will want to know about research concerning weight reduction, the documentation of the WHY Program itself, and various nutrition plans, and may ask about your experience, qualifications, and past successes in helping others reduce their girth.

- An experimenting person will want to approach weight management on a "let me find out what works for me," trial-and-error basis.

Self-Reliance (Frame of Reference)

To elicit a client's frame of reference, ask, "When you've done a good job on something, how do you know? Do you prefer feedback from others, or do you rely more on your own opinion?"

- People who "sort by others" are likely to heed the opinions and advice of people they respect, including you. They are motivated by approval, and sometimes crushed by disapproval or criticism. Your feedback and praise will be meaningful to such clients, so choose your words carefully. When they aren't sure of a course of action, ask, "What have you heard other people advise?" or "What do you think your friends and loved ones would want for you?" People who rely on external validation face the challenge of fairly judging their own efforts in the absence of feedback from others.

- People who are more self-reliant are likely to abide by their own counsel. Your feedback and praise may seem appreciated and accepted, but it is less consequential than the person's own personal assessment. Sometimes internally validating people are overly critical of themselves or, conversely, sometimes they tend to overlook their own mistakes. Hearing about the experiences of others does not convince them to take action.

Sociability

One way to identify where a client falls on the sociability continuum is to ask, "When you are working on a project, do you generally like to work by yourself or with others?"

- For clients who like to pursue projects alone, don't suggest group activities, such as exercise classes or support groups. These folks are not joiners. They like to work at their own pace and do things their own way.

- More sociable clients, who enjoy group activities, might feel more motivated if they join clubs, attend classes, and pursue their weight reduction plans on the "buddy system."

Direction of Motivation

When the client gives his or her reasons for reducing weight, is the motivation mainly "toward" or "away from"?

- Give clients who are motivated "toward" kudos, praise, and compliments. Build in rewards and incentives for success—a small refund, a gift, or a discount coupon for a therapeutic massage or an image consultation (you can usually obtain these from colleagues who offer the services). Help these clients stay motivated by focusing on their sense of accomplishment and the rewards of achieving their weight reduction goals.

- Remind "away from" clients of the health and social consequences of excess weight. Remind them that they want to avoid repeating the frustrations and disappointments of past failures in achieving their weight reduction goals.

Options or Procedures

Does your client prefer to follow rules and procedures or to go with the flow, being spontaneous and open to new possibilities? This distinction speaks to his or her degree of flexibility.

- Most weight reduction programs work better for clients who like to follow rules and procedures. For these clients, emphasize that the route to success is through careful planning of meals, scheduling exercise, following their doctor's recommendations, completing the assignments, and adhering to the "rules" of the WHY Program.

- Clients who like spontaneity and flexibility soon get bored with a routine. Encourage them to find creativity and variety in meal planning and in their exercise program. Support these clients in taking responsibility for working through the program at their own pace. Welcome their input into the structure and process for each session.

Global versus Detail

To find out the client's level of focus, ask, "When you are learning something new for the first time, do you like to start with the details and work up to the big picture, or do you like an overview or outline first?"

- Most people process information by getting the big picture first, then by working down to the details. Your best opening gambit is to present an overview or outline, and then fill in the details.

- The rare detail person is very astute about details but may lose sight of the larger purpose. Appreciate that a detail person wants to conceptualize goals and outcomes in detail. It isn't enough to say, "Eat a healthy diet." Specify what constitutes a healthy diet and how a healthy diet is part of a larger program that leads to specific rewards.

With practice you can leverage Meta-Programs to enhance your client's motivation and determination over time. For more information on Meta-Programs, I recommend two additional books: *Words That Change Minds* (Charvet 1995) and *Figuring Out People* (Bodenhamer and Hall 1997a).

Metaphors and Analogies

If you are creative in storytelling, consider therapeutic metaphors and analogies that convey messages about the importance of various aspects of proper nutrition and exercise. An analogy is a statement that makes a comparison between two things, such as "eating junk food is like turning your body into a garbage disposal," or "having excess weight is like wearing a parka on a ninety-degree day." A therapeutic metaphor is a story that contains a message to the client—a "moral of the story." Analogies and metaphors can orient a client's thinking in new directions.

Here are the advantages of therapeutic metaphors:

- A message conveyed through a captivating story may be more easily received and remembered than direct advice. A message delivered in a metaphor may also bypass a client's conscious resistance to a new idea (Gordon 1978).

- A well-crafted metaphor allows the client to develop his or her own interpretations of the message in the story. According to Lankton and Lankton (1983), metaphors create a "trans-derivational search" process in which the listener searches for the meaning of the metaphor within for her or her own associations and memories. Lankton (1990, p. 1) has said of metaphors, "Change does not result from the flow of the story line, story content, or story outcome. Change results from the retrieving and linking of experience."

- A well-told metaphor can be hypnotic and trance-inducing, serving as a medium for embedded suggestions, hypnotic language patterns, installing anchors and strategies, attribution and indirect communication, and reframing.

- Metaphors suggest changes for which the client can take credit, thus fostering independence.

The best metaphors contain an indirect parallel to the client's situation and echo the wording the client uses in describing problems, dilemmas, desired outcomes, and resources. An example: For a compulsive eater who wants "freedom" from sugar cravings, you could devise a story about a prisoner who hates the confines of prison, detests eating the same food day after day, and longs for freedom, and eventually gets paroled and finds a way to become a law-abiding citizen.

Constructing a Therapeutic Metaphor

You may choose to tell your stories within the context of a conversation or while the client is in a formally induced trance. Deliver the story in an engaging manner. To construct a therapeutic metaphor, follow these steps:

1. Decide on the main message of the metaphor. The message should help the client think in different ways about the problem at hand and should be linked to his or her desired outcome.

2. Create the central figure(s) of the metaphor. The protagonist should be a character with whom the client can identify. The protagonist could be a person, a group of people, an animal, a mythical figure, or perhaps even an inanimate object that is personified. The protagonist faces a challenge that represents the client's overriding problem. The protagonist, for example, may have to solve a puzzle, face an enemy, negotiate a danger or risk, acquire a skill, struggle with a choice, rectify a wrong, undergo a process of learning and transformation, seize an opportunity, or perhaps perform a heroic deed. Other characters in the metaphor can represent significant people in the client's environment or traits or ego states within the client. Do not make yourself a central character in the metaphor, as to do so might seem self-serving.

3. Embellish the story with descriptions and dialogue to make the characters come to life. Create vivid word-pictures and give the story drama to evoke emotions in the listener. You can activate curiosity with the elements of double entendre, confusion, mystery, suspense, and surprise. Add just enough detail to capture the listener's attention and spark the imagination.

4. Create a series of events in the story that bring the characters into action. Carry the story through to a conclusion.

You can find handy metaphors in fairy tales, fables, folktales, myths, ballads, songs, poems, television shows, novels, and movies. One of my favorite fairy tales is the story of the "ugly duckling" who discovers "the truth about herself": she is not a duck at all, but a beautiful swan. You can maintain a collection of general-purpose metaphors for common problems your clients present, and tailor the stories to each individual client. Your metaphors might have happy endings, or you might tell cautionary tales that carry unhappy endings for characters who behave badly. What would have been the fate of Cinderella if she had gone to the ball and just hung out at the buffet eating all the goodies, instead of dancing with the handsome prince?

Lankton and Lankton (1983) give guidance on creating embedded metaphors, or stories within stories, structured in the manner practiced by Dr. Milton H. Erickson. Embedded metaphors can stimulate curiosity and create multiple learning opportunities because of their layered structure. The embedded metaphor consists of three stories around complementary themes. Deliver the embedded metaphor in this way, making a conversational segue between each step:

1. Begin story 1 and stop halfway through it.
2. Begin story 2 and stop halfway through it.
3. Begin story 3 and stop halfway through it.
4. Deliver direct suggestions: "As you are listening to this story, I wonder if you are asking yourself, 'How is it possible that someone can, _____ [insert client's name], change an old belief?'"
5. Conclude story 3.
6. Conclude story 2.
7. Conclude story 1.

Milton H. Erickson frequently used teaching stories based around universal experiences such as learning a skill, retrieving resources from the past, solving a difficult problem, transforming a weakness into an asset, or paying attention to one thing while ignoring another. Common metaphorical themes for clients with weight issues might be these:

* changing the belief that being fat is a means of protection
* changing the belief that food is a way to soothe emotional difficulties
* expressing fear and anger more directly, rather than by being fat
* resisting temptation; saying no and meaning it
* making choices and decisions
* forgoing an immediate, short-lived gain for a longer-term, more meaningful outcome

- learning to apply motivation, determination, discipline, and persistence in pursuit of a goal
- valuing and comforting oneself in new ways
- feeling empowered and confident
- acquiring new coping skills and countering self-sabotage
- creating new meanings and associations around food, exercise, and self.

Finally, listen for any metaphor themes your clients give you from their own experiences and internal maps. Your client might say, "I sometimes think of doughnuts as my only friends at work." You might then offer a story about friends who prove to be enemies, or about learning to choose better friends. If a client says, "My weight shields me from taking risks," you might then tell a story about a knight who was so weighed down by his armor, heavy sword, and over-large shield that he was consistently beaten in battle by more nimble opponents.

Here is a story for people who say they derive comfort from binging on sweets:

> I remember I once had a friend, Betsy, who was a single mom with a cute little girl, Hannah, about three years old. One day when the two were out together for a walk in the park, the little girl slipped and skinned her knee and, of course, she wailed so loudly that strangers nearby turned to look. Betsy felt embarrassed by all the commotion and quickly went to a vendor on the curb and bought a chocolate cookie to soothe the little girl. Little did Betsy realize she was teaching her daughter that chocolate equals comfort.
>
> Another day, Hannah drew a picture and showed it to her mommy. Her mommy was very busy and didn't take the time to sit with Hannah and admire the artwork. Instead, she said, "Thank you, Hannah. What a sweet picture. Here, have a chocolate cookie for being such a good little girl. Now run along." I wonder if Hannah got the idea that chocolate equals reward.
>
> I did hear that one day, while unsupervised, Hannah climbed up on the kitchen counter, balancing precariously on the back of a chair, and got the chocolate cookies out of the cupboard. Like most little kids, she probably thought to herself, "If one cookie is good, more is better." So Hannah ate the whole sack of cookies and got a terrible stomachache and threw up all those cookies—imagine all that chocolate vomit!
>
> Later, in the emergency room, the doctor told Betsy that Hannah was getting too many sweets. He said, "_____, [Insert client's name.] you need to cut back on those cookies and sweets." Betsy said, "But if I deprive her, she will cry and throw temper tantrums. I just can't stand it!" The wise old doctor smiled and said gently, "You are the grown-up in charge. You can say no, and when you give her your attention instead of cookies, she won't feel deprived at all." I guess it

pays to pay attention to what children really want and notice what we teach them inadvertently.

Delivering a Therapeutic Metaphor

Here are some tips on delivering a metaphor:

1. Tell your story with confidence, adding drama and flair though your facial expressions, the pace of your delivery, meaningful pauses, expressive voice tone and pitch, and gestures. You might even employ visual aids.

2. When telling the story, watch the client's nonverbal responses and pace the story accordingly. If, for example, you see a look of surprise on the client's face, you could insert, "Like you, I was surprised myself when I heard about it."

3. When your metaphor is finished, don't give a detailed explanation of its meaning. You can deliver the "moral" and leave it at that. For example, you might say, "So you see, _____ [insert client's name], it is possible for even a coward to be courageous, under the right circumstances." Let your listener decide how the story applies to his or her own life. Just segue to another subject and continue with the session.

Languaging the Past and Present

Clients come to practitioners because they want a solution to a problem. They experience the problem as "here and now." Their representation of the solution, if they have one at all, is that it exists somewhere in the not-so-accessible future. You can change their thinking dramatically simply by changing verb tense. Talk about the problem as though it were in the past—as something the client has done. Talk about the behaviors, feelings, and thoughts that lead to the outcome as though they are already ongoing.

People stay "stuck" in their problem behaviors because they represent those behaviors as continuously in the "now." Sometimes they even "language" their difficulties into the future, predicting that the difficulties are bound to continue unabated, as in this example:

> **Client:** I just eat too much, whether I am hungry or not. I'll get up from supper feeling full, and then an hour later, I'll be back in the kitchen, looking for something to eat.

You can pace with the client's assertion, "language" the problem into the past, and pose another outcome in the present, leading the client's thinking in a new direction. Here's how:

> **Practitioner:** What has been going on until now is that you were eating when you weren't even hungry. You got up from supper, feeling full, and then you headed back to the kitchen, looking for something to eat. And now you want to change that pattern and do something different. Is that right?

The shift is to describe the problem behavior in past tense, and add "past-laden" words ("then," "previously," "formerly"). Then talk about the solution in the present tense. Here is another example. Notice how the word "but" is juxtaposed next to "gave up" to negate the idea of giving up.

> **Client:** I don't like to exercise. I know I should, but I'll try it for a few days, and then just give up on it. It never works for me.

> **Practitioner:** In the past, when you tried to exercise, you didn't get much enjoyment out of it, and you felt discouraged. Previously, you gave up, but now, I'm hearing that you want to find a way to make exercise work for you so that it is enjoyable and worthwhile.

When clients describe the thoughts, behaviors, feelings, and outcomes they want in the future, talk about those things as though they are already happening. Just use present tense verbs that make those future behaviors much more real and accessible.

> **Client:** I'll do better this week. I plan to drink water instead of soft drinks.

> **Practitioner:** Good! So this week you are drinking water instead of soft drinks. Now that you have this change in place, you are really moving toward a healthier weight.

Now have the client imagine being in the future, looking back at the change that has already taken place. This tactic reflects Erickson's pseudo-orientation in time (Andreas 1992).

> **Practitioner:** Imagine how you are feeling two weeks from now when you look back and realize how much more energy you have now, since you've been drinking water the entire time, instead of soft drinks.

Read these two sentences:

> Next week you will walk a quarter-mile each morning.

versus

This coming week you are walking a quarter-mile each morning.

Which one is more compelling? Moving future actions into the present makes them easier to visualize. They seem closer on the timeline. Recasting a verb in the present progressive rather than future tense ("you are walking," versus "you will walk") makes it easier for the listener to visualize the verb as a real action. When describing an outcome, describe it in the present tense as often as possible. Avoid the verb "will" because it pushes activity into the future, where it seems less real to the subconscious mind.

Solution-Oriented Questions

Solution-oriented questions presuppose the existence of a solution to a problem. When you are discussing problems and solutions with a client, the way you pose the question helps the client either move toward the solution or stay stuck in the problem.

Suppose the client says, "My problem is that when I feel bored or tired, I eat cookies compulsively, and I can't stop until the whole package is gone." You could offer any number of responses. Compare these two:

What have you thought about when you've felt bored or tired?

versus

What is a healthy alternative to coping with feeling bored or tired by eating?

Both questions are legitimate responses, depending on where you want the dialogue to go. The first question asks for more information about the problem. The second question focuses directly on the solution and gets the client thinking about a new outcome. Solution-oriented questions can come in handy for keeping both you and the client focused on the outcome. They are especially helpful at the end of a session. Here are a few more solution-oriented questions you may want to use:

What one thing can you do this week that moves you closer to your target weight?

How are you making sure you are eating low-calorie foods while on vacation?

How often are you getting on the skiing machine this week?

How can you stay active, if the rain prevents you from taking a walk?

How are you working things out with your husband so he watches the baby while you go for a walk?

What are some tactful ways to decline when your grandmother offers you her homemade chocolate cake?

What is a better way to cope with stress?

How are you keeping track of calories this coming week?

How can we work together more effectively so that you are really moving toward your outcomes?

How do you plan to celebrate when the first ten pounds have come off?

How do you think it feels to wear a size 8 again?

Summary

What specific strategies in this chapter do you most want to remember and put to use in your conversations with clients?

After all, it's not about whether you found this chapter hard or easy, but about whether you can have fun with these patterns and use them effectively to help clients.

By the way, you don't *have* to learn all these patterns at once. You could appreciate the overall purpose of this chapter, and then learn the patterns in little bits and small bites. It's like eating a rich chocolate cake. You can enjoy seeing and smelling the entire cake as it comes from the oven, and admire how the cook spreads on the frosting. Then, when it's time for dessert, you can savor a small bite at a time and really enjoy it. Then go away for a while and let that bite digest. Look forward to returning later for another bite that tastes equally delicious, if not more so.

Weight reduction and learning persuasive communication skills are both like cultivating a garden. You plot out what you want to plant and what plants you want to grow where, and then you take it one step at a time. First, you clear the ground. Then you plant the seeds. You water and fertilize. Then, when the sprouts come up, you tend them and protect them until they grow big and strong, yielding ripe vegetables or fresh blossoms, ready to pick and enjoy.

When you consider the information in this chapter, are you developing rules to follow or considering creative options for applying advanced language patterns? Are you more motivated by the possibility of enhancing your communication skills or of avoiding mistakes? Are you visualizing how you can apply these skills, practicing saying some of them aloud, getting a feel for them, or allowing them to become a part of your inner dialogue? Does it improve your learning to share the information with others and get their feedback, or do you prefer to evaluate your progress based on your own experience?

Perhaps while you were reading this chapter you doubted whether you could remember all these language patterns, but now you begin to feel certain you understand them more thoroughly.

Imagine a future date at which you are using advanced language patterns effectively, and only then realizing how much you have already learned.

Chapter 18

Suggestions for Follow-up Sessions

Clients who have completed the WHY Program may want to return to your office or clinic for follow-up sessions and additional work. This chapter contains suggestions on the types of follow-up sessions you might offer or recommend.

Self-Esteem Issues

Certainly, self-esteem is an issue for many overweight and formerly overweight individuals. Low self-esteem and obesity are often linked to childhood abuse or emotional neglect as a result of which food became a means of medicating emotions and excess weight took on many unconscious meanings and began serving unconscious purposes. Some clients may find it useful to attend additional sessions to work through the trauma and aftermath of abuse, neglect, or dysfunctional family dynamics.

Even as clients begin to see the excess pounds drop off, they may still retain the beliefs and identity of a "fat person." Self-esteem issues may include thoughts and beliefs about one's desirability to potential partners, ability to assert oneself, social inclusion and exclusion, attractiveness, lovability, and self-confidence.

Bandler and Grinder (1979, p. 99) once wrote, "If you've always been fat, you were never chosen to be on a sports team; you were never asked to dance in high school; you never ran fast." The newly slender person may continue to view the world through past experiences of rejection and resentment. Additional therapy can help the client resolve the issues of the past that fostered low self-esteem, and find new ways to elevate and enhance self-esteem.

Belief Change

Clients may want follow-up sessions to change beliefs other than those about self-esteem and identity. They may want to address beliefs about personal control over emotions and behaviors, as well as about coping skills; relationships; and competencies in managing food, eating, and exercise patterns.

For example, I once had a female client who kept regaining weight because she believed if she were slender, others (including potential male partners) would like her only because she was physically attractive, while devaluing her talents and personality. Her belief was that if people saw her as attractive, they would not notice her "inner spirit." While doing some belief-change work with her, I reminded her that the body is the temple of the soul. With that one remark, her belief changed. Her dilemma was no longer an either-or proposition. She realized that she could be physically attractive and still be loved and valued for her talents and personality as well.

Body Image Issues

People who achieve their target weight have a new body shape to contend with. Although they may enjoy feeling more agile and attractive, they may also contend with unanticipated fears and sensitivity about their body image. They may not know how to respond to compliments. They may have little or no experience with certain kinds of physical movements, such as dancing or navigating a crowded room. Women, in particular, may be unaccustomed to receiving appreciative glances or flirtatious remarks from men. Some newly slender individuals may not be sure how to dress for their new body size, or how to walk or how to sit. They may still think of themselves as "fat" and feel unsure of themselves while moving through the world in a different-sized body. Again, therapy and counseling can help in numerous ways, through modified perceptions, mirror work, and accessing states of confidence and assertiveness.

Relationship Concerns

For some, weight reduction brings a change in social relationships. Be prepared to help your clients process their feelings about such changes and make decisions about how they choose to handle those changes. For example, it may be challenging to some clients when friends and family express amazement about their change in appearance. "You are so handsome (or beautiful) now" may seem to imply "You were so ugly before" or "I told you so" or "Why didn't you do this a long time ago?" Perhaps even worse may be the situation where friends and family express pessimism that the weight reduction will last: "How long do you think you'll keep it off this time?"

The client's newfound attractiveness may upset the dynamics of a relationship with a spouse or significant other who feels jealous or wants reassurance that the relationship is secure. When the client's spouse is overweight as well, the tenor of the relationship will undoubtedly change, as the spouse who is still obese may feel pressure to "catch up" or may feel the loss of a "binge buddy."

Losing weight may also affect friendships. Friendships built around "how tough it is to be fat" or "how diets never work for us" or "how great it is to get together and eat all those luscious, fattening foods," are sure to change. Ambivalence is an understandable response for a formerly overweight individual who no longer feels comfortable with friends who are overweight. Additionally, a young person who has lost weight may have mixed feelings about being newly included in whatever the "in" crowd happens to be. Imagine how a formerly overweight person feels upon hearing derisive comments about fat people—they can still sting!

Communication Skills

Some people "hide" behind fat to avoid confronting others or verbally expressing anger. They may use being overweight as a passive way to say no to others. Once those extra pounds are gone, your clients may benefit from counseling and coaching in assertive communication, negotiation, and conflict-resolution skills.

Self-Motivation Skills

Changing longstanding habits is one achievement. Maintaining those changes year after year is another. Many people who come to counseling and therapy just don't have conscious strategies for making lasting changes. They don't know how to keep motivating themselves, how to instill discipline in themselves, or how to convince themselves to stick to a commitment and a plan, regardless of distractions, setbacks, or transient emotions. Teach your clients how to motivate themselves to stay on track.

Resources

You can consult any number of NLP texts for methods to help clients with these issues. I particularly recommend Hall and Belknap's *The Sourcebook of Magic* (2004). For identity issues, consider Hall's Dis-Identification Pattern in that text. For belief-change work, you could use the Submodality Belief Change Pattern or Dilts' Reimprinting Pattern (Dilts 1990), or Dilts' Walking Belief Change Pattern (McDonald 1979). The Six-Step Reframe and Visual Squash Pattern (Bandler and Grinder 1982) are also good ways to change limiting beliefs.

For relationship skills, consider perceptual shifts and Connirae Andreas' perceptual alignment patterns (Andreas and Andreas 1991). For motivating clients to make lasting changes, I favor timeline work (see James and Woodsmall 1988; Bodenhamer and Hall 1997b) and core transformation, developed by Andreas and Andreas (1994). For resolving past trauma, use visual-kinesthetic dissociation (Andreas or Andreas 1989) or eye movement integration (Beaulieu 2003). For other issues, consider NLP patterns such as new behavior generator, Meta-States Patterns, submodalities work, guided imagery, metaphor, and change personal history processes.

Chapter 19

Tough Questions and Answers about the WHY Program

In chapter 5 I listed several ideas for marketing the WHY Program. You may have noticed something about the suggestions: many of them require that you speak knowledgably about the program. Speaking knowledgably may entail answering some tough questions about the WHY Program. To help you answer those questions, I've dedicated this chapter to the toughest questions about the program I have encountered and the answers I give.

Q: Is the WHY Program safe?

A: Yes. Safety was one of the chief considerations in developing this program. Every client is advised to have a physical examination prior to enrolling in the program. Additionally, clients are advised to follow a physician-approved nutrition and exercise plan tailored to individual health needs. I regularly refer my clients to other health specialists such as nutritionists, physical trainers, and psychiatrists.

Hypnosis, when practiced by a trained, qualified mental-health professional, has been proven safe and effective in helping people lose weight, with no physical side-effects. Research studies recommend hypnotherapy as an adjunct to medically supervised weight reduction programs built around nutritional planning and exercise (see appendix A: "Abstracts of Studies on Hypnotherapy for Weight Control").

Q: How does the WHY Weight Reduction Program work?

A: The program focuses on the cognitive-behavioral elements of weight control that are most directly related to success or failure in weight reduction. These elements are stress management; food selection; and adherence to a good nutrition plan, portion control, healthy eating patterns, and exercise. Additionally, the program indirectly addresses secondary issues such as personal responsibility, self-nurturance, positive thinking and self-talk, self-imposed obstacles, and motivation.

Q: Is the WHY Program appropriate for any client who is overweight?

A: No, this program is not for any or every client with weight issues. The practitioner follows guidelines for accepting each client, and has been advised as to medical and clinical contraindications. In general, the program is not recommended for clients who have other serious health problems that need more immediate attention or who have medical issues that might interfere with weight reduction. The program is not for clients who are pregnant or breastfeeding. It is not recommended for clients in a major life crisis or for those who are impaired due to psychotic disorders or active abuse of alcohol or illegal or prescription drugs.

The program was not designed for children or for people who are cognitively challenged or impaired. Teens may participate in the program, provided they have motivation and full parental permission, support, and supervision. The WHY Program is contraindicated for teens who are presenting other issues such as acting out, delinquency, truancy, drug and alcohol use, or depression. The program is not recommended for adults who would do well to obtain treatment for other current issues such as relationship problems, criminal activity, occupational misconduct, trauma or abuse, active grief, depression, or psychotic behavior.

The WHY Program is not recommended for individuals who maintain unrealistic expectations about weight reduction, have not consulted a physician about their weight-control issues, or do not wish to comply with program instructions. Practitioners should exercise clinical judgment and caution when offering the WHY Program to individuals who are elderly, have physical disabilities, or have a history of anorexia or bulimia. The practitioner consults with the client's primary-care physician before conducting any weight reduction program with these types of individuals.

Q: This program does not directly address underlying issues such as self-esteem, childhood traumas, or possible previous abuse—might these be related to compulsive eating?

A: Yes, such issues are often related to compulsive eating, and most practitioners are aware of this probability. Although most practitioners agree that in many cases obesity is the result of such underlying issues, most consumers of mental-health services do not think that way. In our society it is much more acceptable for a client to seek therapy for overeating than for childhood abuse, trauma, or low self-esteem. Clients rarely attribute their weight problems to such underlying causes. In addition, some clients have been in therapy for months or even years to address issues of self-esteem, trauma, and abuse, but remain overweight nevertheless.

Clients often attribute their weight problems to difficulty managing stress, inability to eat moderately, inability to determine when they feel full, and uncontrollable compulsions to eat. Moreover, some clients would argue that it is difficult to maintain self-esteem while knowingly engaging in unhealthy behaviors and seeing themselves as unattractive and fat. An improved appearance and healthier behaviors sometimes lead to an enhanced sense of personal pride and self-acceptance, and a willingness to get additional therapy.

Clinicians and practitioners are advised to carefully screen clients who apply for the WHY Program, and to exercise caution about enrolling clients who are severely dysfunctional, depressed, or personality disordered. Practitioners also advise clients, when appropriate, that deeper emotional issues could be the root cause of obesity and that, if left untreated, such issues could lead to self-sabotage. Clinicians are advised (a) to offer such clients treatment for underlying issues (if qualified to do so), or (b) to refer them to other professionals who specialize in issues such as depression, childhood abuse, trauma, or low self-esteem.

If a client wants to enroll in the WHY Program after completing therapy for underlying issues, then again, the practitioner should evaluate whether the client is functioning at an appropriate level of mental and emotional stability. The evaluation criteria should screen for symptoms that the client displayed previously, according to the client's previous diagnosis. These symptoms might include suicide ideation, self-mutilation or similar behaviors, night terrors, drinking binges, startle responses, panic attacks, anger-management problems, promiscuity, inability to form and maintain friendships, obsessive-compulsive behaviors, or participation in dysfunctional and abusive relationships.

The WHY Program is appropriate for individuals who have successfully undergone therapy for deeper issues and now need help establishing an intelligent relationship with food and in developing healthy eating and exercise habits.

Q: Who is qualified to conduct the WHY Program?

A: The program is designed for administration by medical personnel, certified coaches, and licensed mental-health therapists who are certified in hypnotherapy and Neuro-Linguistic Programming. Practitioners should also have a basic working knowledge of how the body burns calories, healthy weight reduction measures, appropriate weight ranges, the components of healthy nutrition, and weight reduction resources, such as weight-loss programs, facilities, books, and diets.

Q: What should practitioners do about clients who cannot be hypnotized?

A: Assuming that hypnotizability, like most human traits, follows the bell curve distribution, most individuals can be hypnotized to some degree. People are amenable to hypnosis under these conditions:

- They want to be hypnotized.
- They expect good results from hypnosis.
- They have a good rapport with the hypnotherapist.
- The hypnotherapist has cleared all their concerns and answered their questions.

Practitioners have the option of conducting some initial tests of hypnotizability with clients who have no formal experience with hypnosis. For the rare candidate who does not respond well to hypnosis, the practitioner may opt to delay the remaining WHY Program sessions and spend an extra session teaching the client how to feel comfortable and relaxed with the hypnosis process.

Hypnotizability often improves once the practitioner has answered the client's questions and concerns, and provided reassurance that hypnosis is a safe, often pleasant experience. Practitioners are also prepared to tailor their hypnotic approaches to each client's individual needs, whenever possible, ethical, and practical. If, after all this, the client still cannot be hypnotized, then the practitioner could discontinue the program and refer the client to another hypnotherapist who might have a better rapport with the client or who might offer a different approach to which the client is more amenable.

Q: Does the WHY Program really work?

A: This after all, is the ultimate question for all therapeutic work, isn't it? No program is worth the time and expense involved if it does not work. When I investigated the question, I found that the answer was not straightforward. The most honest answer I can give is, "It depends." Allow me to elaborate.

First, no weight reduction program has a 100 percent success rate. In fact, most weight programs work for some participants but not for others. Every kind of weight reduction program has participants who give up, drop out, lose interest, or regain the weight they lost. If weight reduction programs were universally successful, we'd see a decrease in the number of people who are overweight—instead, those numbers have increased over the past two decades, despite numerous new diets, studies, and information about the causes and dangers of obesity.

It has been my experience with the WHY Program (especially in the beginning when I was first developing it) that some participants do drop out. Other participants lose weight but do not reach their target weight. Upon encountering these problems, I have modified and improved the program accordingly. With these improvements in the program, more clients have completed the program and are continuing to reach their weight reduction goals.

Second, participants in any weight reduction program are likely to be easily discouraged and to drop out of the program, even when they have paid in advance, due to a variety of factors:

- depression around stressful life events that occur over the course of the program
- lack of strategies for maintaining resilience and motivation over time
- a host of chronic health problems that accompany obesity, particularly in individuals over age forty

For these reasons, it is essential that practitioners follow these three guidelines:

- Carefully screen clients for the program (see chapter 3).
- During the initial session, obtain a congruent commitment from the client to comply with program requirements (see chapter 6).
- Give extra encouragement, persuasion, and coaching to clients who seem stuck, are having difficulty fulfilling the requirements of the program, or may be tempted to drop out of the program (see chapter 15).

If practitioners follow these guidelines, program participants are more likely to achieve success and have a satisfying experience with the program.

The WHY Program does result in weight reduction for clients who complete the eight sessions. Listening to the recordings seems to be an important factor. A few people even return for additional counseling. One woman, for example, felt so much more energized and confident upon reducing by the initial sixteen pounds that she returned for sessions on how to excel in her business endeavors. As evidence of the efficacy of the WHY Program, here are comments and testimonials from satisfied clients. These remarks are documented here with client permission and anonymity.

> My association with you seems to keep me on track, whereas in the past, usually at ninety days into a diet, I lose interest and I give up. It seems there is some inner force guiding me and pushing me this time that is different.
> —G. J. (reduced 16 pounds by eighth session)

I hear your voice in my mind. It's self-talk that wasn't there before. Now when I look at some fattening food in the store—like one day it was fried chicken and another day it was carrot cake—some food I shouldn't eat, I say to myself, "You don't need that."

—P. M. (reduced 14 pounds by eighth session)

What I appreciated was the tapes. They helped me change my outlook. Weight control will always be a lifelong thing for me, but I do things differently now. For example, I now walk my dog for a mile every day. The program put me on a schedule. I needed that structure. It was wonderful. The one thing I learned: if you can control your mind, with a focus on the goal, that's the trick. The sessions were very relaxing, like a mini-vacation. It was so pleasant.

—J. B. (reduced 45 pounds over the year
following participation)

You know, I can't explain exactly how [but] I just didn't want sweets and fattening food any more, and I am eating less. I didn't exercise much before, but now I walk at least twice a week. People are amazed at the change and, of course, I'm more sociable and confident. If I think I'm starting to slip back into old habits, I listen to the tapes or remember the things we talked about. I never knew I could make so many changes in my life just by changing my thinking.

—J. L. (reduced 20 pounds over the year
following participation)

I wanted a long-term weight-loss and weight-management program. This one fit my needs perfectly. I appreciated that Dr. Pearson modified each session to meet my particular desires.

—R. F. (reduced 70 pounds over the year
following participation)

I wanted to gain control of my poor eating habits and get on track to better health. Also, I needed to deal with stress in my life. My stress load … has been greatly reduced. I'm now able to focus on healthy choices in my diet. I have control of my life back! This work is so valuable to me that I will refer others. I wish I knew about this program years ago.

—A. G. (reduced 45 pounds over the year
following participation)

The number of sessions was just right. I wanted to change my eating habits, and to a great extent, I have. In fact, I waited one month after the program was done to give this testimonial, to see if the changes would "stick" without the sessions. They have and I have lost more pounds! The work was outstanding. I came in with skepticism. I felt more confident after the first session.

—G. B. (reduced 18 pounds by eighth session)

Somehow there's been a force that has got me where I am. I haven't lost this much weight before, and I'm still eager and energetic to lose more weight and get back into shape, in spite of health problems. I haven't lost interest. I do not get discouraged. I just stick with it. In the past, I've never been able to maintain the focus and concentration to stay with it this long, and it's been eight months. I attribute this to the suggestions that are now in my subconscious mind.

—B. J. (reduced 17 pounds by eighth session)

Chapter 20

Final Thoughts on Addictions and Compulsive Eating

An Interview with Jon Connelly, Ph.D. L.C.S.W.

Have you ever sat with a master practitioner and found yourself spellbound by the stories and the conversation that answered your questions in ways you didn't expect? That's what happened for me on a sunny morning in July 2005, when I had the privilege to interview Dr. Jon Connelly about his innovative approaches to working with addictions and compulsive eating.

Jon specializes in clinical hypnosis and rapid trauma resolution. He is the founder and director of the Institute for Survivors of Sexual Violence, Inc., a not-for-profit corporation located in Jupiter, Florida. He has more than thirty years of experience working with emotional, behavioral, sexual, and relationship problems; supervising mental-health professionals; and conducting nationally recognized training programs in advanced psychotherapeutic methods. His training programs for mental-health practitioners focus on advanced methods for treating problem anger, protracted grieving, anxiety, depression, and psychological trauma. He has produced two training manuals for his students, entitled *Life Change Conversations: The Power of Transformational Communication* and *Dynamic Hypnotherapy & Rapid Trauma Resolution.*

Appeal, Possibility, Priority, and Conflict

Jon's insightful approach to addictions and compulsive eating begins with examining four basic elements of behavioral change.

> It's advantageous to examine four things. One, is the outcome appealing to the individual? Two, is the outcome possible, and does the individual fully realize it is possible? Three, is it a priority? Four, is there a conflict with either the outcome itself or getting there? With weight control, some people might be willing to do those things that would be necessary to accomplish the result, but have some conflict about being slim and attractive. Other individuals have no conflict with being slim and attractive but have conflict about doing what's necessary to reach the desired outcome.
>
> Here's an example. A lady told me she had a strong desire to lose weight. She was about twenty pounds overweight. She was happily married, and she was

frequently entertaining and throwing parties for her husband's business associates. What happened when she would start to lose weight [was that] she began to look more and more sexually attractive. She told me, "When I have these parties, people are happy to see me, and they give me a big hug when they see me. When I lose weight, the hugs are different. They are more sexual." When her husband's friends were coming on to her, she would race out and buy ice cream and start putting on all the weight she'd lost.

Before I worked with her, she was not even conscious of this conflict. All she knew was that every time she would lose weight, she would eat herself back to being overweight. When the fear which caused the conflict was exposed, we were able to eliminate the problem, and she was then able to lose the weight she wanted to lose.

Sometimes people don't do something because other things are a higher priority. In order for behavioral change to take place, it's necessary that the desired change be a higher priority than anything that would compete with it.

I teach people that it is important to ask the right question in order to get the right answer. If someone has eliminated a smoking addiction, it is best not to ask if a cigarette would be enjoyable. The better question would be, "Do I want to become a smoker again?" The question, "Would you enjoy a doughnut?" might get a very different answer from, "Would you like to be off-track, feel out of control, and get fat?"

Some people, and even some practitioners, believe that there is a devilish or evil part of the mind that is tempting the individual to indulge in substances that would be harmful. I view it as a well-intentioned but short-sighted facet of the mind. This part of the mind doesn't see far enough into the future to see the negative effect of a behavior. This childlike facet of the mind should not be the part controlling behavior.

Sometimes, when people have failed to succeed, they believe that they lack the necessary ingredients for success. This can perpetuate a self-fulfilling prophecy that leads to future failure or even prevents any attempt to bring about change. Being stuck has nothing to do with weakness. Resolving the issues that have blocked change will make success possible.

The Language of Change

Sometimes people are stuck because of a language pattern. It is more powerful to tell yourself you want to be slender than it is to tell yourself you need to lose weight. Desire is more powerful than need. Feelings of necessity and obligation deplete joy and energy.

Sometimes people talk about their behaviors as though the behavior is an attribute or an identity. They say, "I'm a smoker." Now, it's about self, rather than about behavior. "It's who I am." When people talk about a problem as "self," then it is so much harder to change the behavior. It is much easier to change your behavior than it is to change your self.

The Point of Choice Is the Present

Jon made it clear that the point of choice is always *now*; always in the present moment:

> It's impossible to do or not do anything in the future, because we don't live in the future. Certainty is available in abundance in the present but becomes scarce as we move our thoughts into the future. You don't have to not smoke or not overeat in the future. All you have to do is not smoke or not overeat *right now*, and that is possible.

> If you aren't eating or smoking right now, then it means you have the ability to refrain from doing it.

Trying and Hoping

> People who desire a behavioral change often use words like "try" or "hope." "Try" tells the subconscious that there is doubt that it can happen. "Hope" is even worse because it tells our mind that we have no say, no power. Instead of trying or hoping, one would be better off using the phrase "I am doing it" to both acknowledge and perpetuate success.

Certainty

> An addictive substance creates a desire for more and more of itself. A craving is the mind asking for something. When there is certainty, there are no cravings. The mind will not ask for what there is no possibility of getting. Certainty provides the ultimate in comfort, because nothing is left to chance.

Thus, I ended my conversation with Dr. Jon Connelly, an amazing hypnotherapist. Somehow that conversation also seems a fitting ending for this book.

Appendixes

Appendix A

Abstracts of Studies on Hypnotherapy for Weight Control

Scientific research shows hypnotherapy to be effective for weight reduction when used in conjunction with behavioral therapy. Studies recommend that an effective hypnotherapy program for weight control consist of six to eight or more sessions of group or individual hypnotherapy. This appendix summarizes representative studies conducted between 1985 and 1998 on the effectiveness of hypnosis in weight control. The abstracts are presented in alphabetical order, according to the last name of the lead author. The findings are also summarized as a report in appendix B.

Allison, D. B., and M. S. Faith. 1996. Hypnosis as an adjunct to cognitive-behavioral psychotherapy for obesity: A meta-analytical appraisal. *Journal of Consulting and Clinical Psychology* **64 (3): 513–16.**
In this meta-analytical examination of clinical weight-loss studies, Allison and Faith examined the effectiveness of hypnosis as an adjunct to cognitive-behavioral psychotherapy. The studies consistently found that hypnotherapy enhanced cognitive-behavioral approaches to weight reduction.

Andersen, M. S. 1985. Hypnotizability as a factor in the hypnotic treatment of obesity. *International Journal of Clinical and Experimental Hypnosis* **33 (2): 150–59.**
Andersen conducted a program of time-limited, relatively uncontaminated hypnotherapy for the treatment of obesity, exploring the relationship between hypnotizability, as measured by the Stanford Hypnotic Susceptibility Scale, form A, and success at weight reduction via self-hypnosis. The participants were 43 outpatients, male and female, ranging in age from 21 to 56, at the Morton Prince Center for Hypnotherapy in New York City. Thirty participants completed the program, which consisted of an orientation session, eight weekly individual treatment sessions, and twelve weeks of follow-up, during which the participants practiced self-hypnosis. The 30 participants who completed the program had an average weight loss of 20.2 pounds. Results indicated a statistically significant positive association between degree of hypnotizability and success at weight reduction. Highly hypnotizable participants did significantly better on the weight reduction program than did participants who scored in the medium to low hypnotizability range.

Barabasz, M., and D. Spiegel. 1989. Hypnotizability and weight loss in obese subjects. *The International Journal of Eating Disorders* 8: 335–41.
Barabasz and Spiegel conducted a controlled study with 45 females, finding that supplementing a basic self-management program for weight loss with hypnosis resulted in slightly increased weight loss at a three-month follow-up.

Bolocofsky, D. N., D. Spinier, and L. Coulthard-Morris. 1985. Effectiveness of hypnosis as an adjunct to behavioral weight management. *Journal of Clinical Psychology* 41 (1): 35–41.
Bolocofsky and colleagues conducted a study to determine the effectiveness of hypnotherapy as a component of behavioral therapy for weight control. The 109 participants, mostly women, ranged in age from 17 to 67 years. The participants were randomly assigned to two different treatment groups, behavioral therapy and hypnotherapy. Within the two groups, the participants were again randomly assigned to specific therapists. The purpose of the behavioral treatments was "to familiarize the participants with their present inappropriate eating habits and to enable them to learn behaviors more conducive to weight loss and maintenance." Each participant began a similar treatment program, with some components personalized for individual specific needs. Nine weekly meetings took place, in which "the emphasis was on slowing down food consumption, recognizing and modifying responses to stimuli that preceded maladaptive eating behaviors, charting weight changes, and developing enduring methods of self-reinforcement for successful weight loss." The hypnosis group followed the same program, except that the rules were given to the participants in the form of hypnotic suggestions, via either self-hypnosis or hypnosis by the therapist. The final results, after follow-ups at eight months and two years, showed that "although both interventions resulted in a significant weight change from the initial to final sessions, only the group that utilized hypnosis continued to lose a significant amount of weight."

Cochrane, G. 1992. Hypnosis and weight reduction: Which is the cart and which is the horse? *American Journal of Clinical Hypnosis* 35 (2): 109–18.
In a review of scientific literature on hypnosis and weight loss, Cochrane concluded that hypnosis can reveal the specific reasons why people overeat and that this realization, in turn, can help therapists prescribe specific interventions targeted at those reasons. Cochrane stated that "hypnosis then, in research, theory, and practice, must be adapted to the problem and perceived not as a treatment but as a potentially valuable aspect of effective treatment."

Cochrane, G., and J. Friesen. 1986. Hypnotherapy in weight loss treatment. *Journal of Consulting and Clinical Psychology* 54: 489–92.
Cochrane and Friesen investigated the effects of hypnosis on weight loss for 60 females, all at least 20 percent overweight. Treatment included group hypnosis with metaphors for ego strengthening, decision making, and motivation, and individual and group hypnosis with maintenance suggestions. The group exposed to hypnosis was more successful than a control group: 17 pounds reduced versus 0.5 pounds at follow-up.

Coman, C., and B. Evans. 1995. Clinical update on eating disorders and obesity: Implications for treatment with hypnosis. *Australian Journal of Clinical and Experimental Hypnosis* **23 (1): 1–13.**
Coman and Evans conducted a review of numerous studies on the effectiveness of hypnotherapy in weight reduction programs. The hypnotherapy methods used in the studies included ego state therapy, age regression, and age progression to identify and correct the origins of participants' disordered cognitions and emotional conflicts associated with eating disorders such as anorexia, bulimia, and compulsive eating. They concluded that hypnotherapy is effective because it addresses faulty cognitions centering on food, identifies eating triggers, and helps with stimulus control.

Farrington, G. 1985. Effects of self-hypnosis audiotapes on weight loss: Relationship with ego-strength, motivation, anxiety, and locus of control. *Dissertation Abstracts International* **46 (6B): 2048.**
In a controlled study, Farrington taught participants to use self-hypnosis audiotapes that promoted mental rehearsal in behavioral change related to weight loss. The study found significant improvement in performance for the treatment groups as compared to the control group.

Greaves, E., G. Tidy, and R. A. S. Christie. 1995. Hypnotherapy and weight loss. *Nutrition and Food Science* **95 (6).**
Greaves, Tidy, and Christie reported on a study of eight participants who were referred from a single general practice. The referral criteria were clinical obesity, lack of success with dieting, and evidence of occupational and social disability due to obesity. Underlying causes of obesity, including endocrine and metabolic factors, were excluded on clinical grounds. One-on-one hypnotherapy was conducted in the general practice surgery environment or in the outpatient unit of the Hitchin Hospital, Hertfordshire, England. All participants showed a limited reduction in basal metabolism index, ranging from 3 percent to 17 percent after hypnotherapy, with progressive weight reduction throughout the course of treatment. A two-year follow-up found that six of the eight patients had maintained a reduced weight, compared to pretreatment. Of these six, four showed a partial relapse but still weighed less than pretreatment.

Kirsch, I., G. Montgomery, and G. Sapirstein. 1995. Hypnosis as an adjunct to cognitive-behavioral weight loss treatments—Another meta-reanalysis. *Journal of Consulting and Clinical Psychology* **63: 214–20.**
Kirsch, Montgomery, and Sapirstein performed a meta-analysis of hypnotic enhancement in cognitive-behavioral weight-loss treatments. The researchers obtained data from two studies and averaged the data across post-treatment and follow-up assessment periods. The mean weight loss was 6.00 pounds without hypnosis and 11.83 pounds with hypnosis. At the last assessment period, the mean weight loss was 6.03 pounds without hypnosis and 14.88 pounds with hypnosis. Analysis indicated that the benefits of hypnosis increased over time.

Schaumberg, L. L., C. A. Patsdaughter, F. K. Selder, and L. Napholz. 1995. Hypnosis as a clinical intervention for weight reduction and self-esteem improvement in young women. *International Journal of Psychiatric Nursing Research* 1 (3): 99–107.

Schaumberg and colleagues, in a controlled clinical trial, found that hypnotherapy was an effective intervention with young women who were treated for both weight problems and low self-esteem.

Stradling, J., D. Roberts, and F. Lovelock. 1998. Controlled trial of hypnotherapy for weight loss in patients with obstructive sleep apnea. *International Journal of Obesity* 22: 278–81.

Stradling, Roberts, and Lovelock examined the efficacy of hypnotherapy in weight loss for 60 obese patients with obstructive sleep apnea. The study took place at a National Health Service hospital in the United Kingdom. The study was a randomized, controlled, parallel study of two forms of hypnotherapy (stress reduction or energy intake reduction) versus dietary advice alone. All three groups lost 2–3 percent of their body weight at three months. At 18 months, only the hypnotherapy group treated with stress reduction still showed a significant but small (3.8 kg) mean weight loss compared to baseline. Analyzed over the whole time period, the hypnotherapy group treated with stress reduction achieved significantly more weight loss than the other two groups, which were not significantly different from each other.

Vanderlinden, J., and W. Vandereycken. 1994. The (limited) possibilities of hypnotherapy in the treatment of obesity. *American Journal of Clinical Hypnosis* 36 (4): 248–57.

Vanderlinden and Vandereycken conducted a review of three controlled, comparative surveys on hypnotherapy in the treatment of obesity and stated that "a combination of behavior therapy and hypnotherapy appeared to produce more weight reduction than a mere behavior therapeutic approach."

Appendix B

Report: Scientific Studies Show Hypnotherapy Can Boost Weight Reduction

More than a decade of controlled scientific studies and analytical reviews show that hypnotherapy, in conjunction with proper exercise and nutrition, can enhance weight reduction and help keep the weight off longer. A review of studies published in leading medical journals between 1985 and 1998 offers compelling evidence that hypnotherapy is the added ingredient that helps people stay on track with weight control.

Here's what the studies found:

- Hypnotherapy is effective in weight reduction when used in conjunction with behavioral therapy.

- Effective hypnotherapy programs generally consist of six to eight or more sessions of group or individual hypnotherapy.

- Study participants who scored highest in hypnotizability had the most significant weight reduction results.

- In studies comparing a control group to a hypnotherapy group, the group exposed to hypnotherapy lost more weight and kept the weight off longer.

- Hypnotherapy helped people correct faulty thinking and associations around food and helped them get control over non-hunger-related eating.

- In a study comparing behavioral therapy to hypnotherapy, both groups of participants showed the same results at the end of the study. At follow-ups at eight months and again at two years, however, only the hypnotherapy group continued to lose weight.

- Hypnotherapy can be administered by a therapist or via hypnosis tapes or self-hypnosis; all three methods proved effective.

- Hypnotherapy helped study participants remember specific weight reduction goals and behavioral recommendations.

- Unlike most programs, which focus only on diet and exercise, hypnotherapy might include suggestions for ego strengthening, decision making, stress management, self-soothing, mental rehearsal, and enhanced motivation, all of which are helpful in successful weight management.

References

Allison, D. B., and M. S. Faith. 1996. Hypnosis as an adjunct to cognitive-behavioral psychotherapy for obesity: A meta-analytical appraisal. *Journal of Consulting and Clinical Psychology* 64 (3): 513–16.

Andersen, M. S. 1985. Hypnotizability as a factor in the hypnotic treatment of obesity. *International Journal of Clinical and Experimental Hypnosis* 33 (2): 150–59.

Barabasz, M., and D. Spiegel. 1989. Hypnotizability and weight loss in obese subjects. *The International Journal of Eating Disorders* 8: 335–41.

Bolocofsky, D. N., D. Spinier, and L. Coulthard-Morris. 1985. Effectiveness of hypnosis as an adjunct to behavioral weight management. *Journal of Clinical Psychology* 41 (1): 35–41.

Cochrane, G. 1992. Hypnosis and weight reduction: Which is the cart and which is the horse? *American Journal of Clinical Hypnosis* 35 (2): 109–18.

Cochrane, G., and J. Friesen. 1986. Hypnotherapy in weight loss treatment. *Journal of Consulting and Clinical Psychology* 54: 489–92.

Coman, C., and B. Evans. 1995. Clinical update on eating disorders and obesity: Implications for treatment with hypnosis. *Australian Journal of Clinical and Experimental Hypnosis* 23 (1): 1–13.

Farrington, G. 1985. Effects of self-hypnosis audiotapes on weight loss: Relationship with ego-strength, motivation, anxiety, and locus of control. *Dissertation Abstracts International* 46 (6B): 2048.

Greaves, E., G. Tidy, and R. A. S. Christie. 1995. Hypnotherapy and weight loss. *Nutrition and Food Science* 95 (6).

Kirsch, I., G. Montgomery, and G. Sapirstein. 1995. Hypnosis as an adjunct to cognitive-behavioral weight loss treatments—Another meta-reanalysis. *Journal of Consulting and Clinical Psychology* 63: 214–20.

Schaumberg, L. L., C. A. Patsdaughter, F. K. Selder, and L. Napholz. 1995. Hypnosis as a clinical intervention for weight reduction and self-esteem improvement in young women. *International Journal of Psychiatric Nursing Research* 1 (3): 99–107.

Stradling, J., D. Roberts, and F. Lovelock. 1998. Controlled trial of hypnotherapy for weight loss in patients with obstructive sleep apnea. *International Journal of Obesity* 22: 278–81.

Vanderlinden, J., and W. Vandereycken. 1994. The (limited) possibilities of hypnotherapy in the treatment of obesity. *American Journal of Clinical Hypnosis* 36 (4): 248–57.

Appendix C

Sample Informed Consent Agreement

The following informed consent agreement is intended simply as an example of such an agreement, which a practitioner can adapt for his or her own purposes. It is not intended as a source of legal authority, advice, or expertise. Practitioners wishing to develop informed consent agreements should consult with their own legal counsel regarding relevant laws and regulations in their jurisdictions.

NAME AND ADDRESS OF YOUR PRACTICE

Weight, Hypnotherapy, and YOU Weight Reduction Program

Informed Consent Agreement

Purpose of This Agreement

This agreement specifies the terms of the business relationship and the therapeutic relationship between NAME OF YOUR PRACTICE (hereafter referred to as Practitioner) and NAME OF CLIENT (hereafter referred to as Client).

Voluntary Consent to Participate

The Client voluntarily consents to participate in the Weight, Hypnotherapy and YOU Weight Reduction Program, provided by NAME OF YOUR PRACTICE. Methods used in this program may include, where appropriate, psychotherapy, counseling, coaching, clinical hypnosis, hypnotherapy, guided imagery, relaxation training, visualization, Neuro-Linguistic Programming, and psychological diagnosis. All such processes are hereafter referred to as "services." The Client agrees to be an active participant in the program and shares responsibility for the process and results. The Client understands and agrees that the Weight, Hypnotherapy and YOU Weight Reduction Program sessions will address only weight reduction and related concerns. The Client agrees to inform the therapist of changes in his/her circumstances or medical status that may adversely affect his/her ability to participate fully in the program.

The Practitioner agrees to render ethical, competent services to the Client, to the best of his/her abilities and within the limits of his/her professional knowledge and training. However, the Client understands that the Practitioner's services are not based on exact science and that results can vary among individuals. The Client understands and agrees that there are NO GUARANTEES as to the results or outcomes. The Client remains ultimately responsible for her/his own decisions, actions, choices, and emotions, during and after participation in the program.

The Client understands and acknowledges that the services to be rendered may consist of a variety of processes and may incorporate questions, visualization, pretending, writing or drawing, role-playing, breathing instructions, eye-movement instructions, take-home assignments, and physical movement. Procedures will be explained to the Client in advance and will be conducted only with the Client's consent. The Client has the right to ask questions about any process and to discuss any concerns before, during, or following these processes. The Client has the right to refuse to participate in any process at any time. The Client has the right to accept or reject instructions, advice, interpretations, or suggestions made by the Practitioner at any time. The Client understands that noncompliance with program instructions may reduce the probability of success.

Limits of Hypnotherapy/Clinical Hypnosis

The Client understands and acknowledges the following: hypnotherapy or clinical hypnosis, like any other form of psychotherapy or counseling, is not an exact science. Hypnotherapy/clinical hypnosis is not a panacea or a magical cure for any ailment or problem. A hypnotherapist has no unusual powers or abilities and merely attempts to communicate so as to facilitate the client's ability to think in a focused manner. The Practitioner makes no claims or guarantees as to the success of hypnotherapy/clinical hypnosis methods, whether the Client will experience trance, or the degree of trance that the Client will experience. There are a number of methods for conducting hypnotherapy, and some methods may be more effective than others with any particular individual. Finding the most helpful method may be a trial-and-error process. Individuals vary as to suggestibility and hypnotizability, and results can be influenced by many factors including the client's personality, motivation, mood, and health.

Hypnotherapy can be relaxing, and some clients may fall asleep or think they have fallen asleep during the process. The Practitioner will, nevertheless, continue the hypnotherapy session, on the assumption that the Client will continue to hear and respond to suggestions and instructions, in the same way that a sleeping person at home will respond to unusual sounds at night. The Client acknowledges that he/she may or may not remember everything the Practitioner says during the hypnotherapy process.

Use of Audio Recordings

As a service to the Client, the Practitioner will make audio recordings of some program sessions, for the Client's possession and use, to reinforce hypnotic approaches to the Client's stated outcomes. Since such recordings include instructions for relaxation, the Client agrees not to play the recordings in a moving vehicle or when operating potentially dangerous equipment. The Client also agrees not to play or listen to the recordings when providing direct supervision to a small child or incapacitated adult. The Client agrees that he/she will not reproduce these audio recordings or use them for commercial purposes or financial gain. Audio recordings produced by NAME OF YOUR PRACTICE are for the Client's personal use. If the Client allows others to listen to audio recordings produced by NAME OF YOUR PRACTICE, then NAME OF YOUR PRACTICE is in no way responsible for outcomes or results, since NAME OF YOUR PRACTICE has not entered into a service contract with any other users or listeners.

Risks

The Client acknowledges that there may be slight risks associated with the Practitioner's services. During the process, the Client may experience some uncomfortable emotions or review some unpleasant memories. The Client may find his/her chosen outcomes difficult to implement. The Client acknowledges that making personal changes in behavior, thinking, and emotions through psychotherapy, counseling, and coaching sometimes requires learning by trial and error and that he/she may make mistakes or experience some confusion or setbacks in the process. The Client acknowledges and accepts these risks.

Confidentiality and Privacy

STATE YOUR POLICIES AND PRACTICES REGARDING CONFIDENTIALITY AND PRIVACY.

Stipulation of Program Parameters

The Client understands that the Weight, Hypnotherapy and YOU Weight Reduction Program consists of eight sessions, equaling INSERT THE NUMBER OF HOURS of face-to-face time with the Practitioner. The Client may also receive written materials with the program. The fee for the entire program must be paid at the time of the first session and is not refundable. The Client understands that after the fourth session, he/she must reduce at least four pounds (two kilos) after each session in order to return for each subsequent session. The Client may end participation at any time he/she chooses to do so, forfeiting remaining sessions and fees.

Referrals to Other Service Providers

It is a condition of participation that the client pursue a medically supervised or physician-approved nutritional program and exercise regimen of his or her choosing, in conjunction with the Weight, Hypnotherapy and YOU Weight Reduction Program. If NAME OF YOUR PRACTICE recommends that the Client seek the services of other service providers, the Client is at liberty to comply with or reject such recommendations. The Client will not hold NAME OF YOUR PRACTICE accountable or liable for the conduct of those care providers to whom the Client is referred.

Clinical Record Keeping and Inspection

STATE YOUR POLICIES REGARDING CLINICAL RECORD KEEPING AND INSPECTION AND THE MANNER IN WHICH RECORDS ARE STORED, MAINTAINED, AND DESTROYED.

STATE YOUR POLICIES AND PRACTICES FOR REPRODUCING AND MAILING COPIES OF CLINICAL RECORDS UPON THE CLIENT'S REQUEST.

Fees

DESCRIBE (A) YOUR FEE STRUCTURE AND THE FEE FOR THE WHY PROGRAM; (B) ANY DISCOUNTS YOU MIGHT OFFER; AND (C) ANY ADDITIONAL CHARGES OR FEES THAT MAY BE INCURRED, SUCH AS FOR POSTAGE, CANCELLATION OF APPOINTMENTS, COPYING RECORDS, OR CHECKS RETURNED FOR INSUFFICIENT FUNDS.

Insurance Coverage

STATE YOUR POLICIES AND PRACTICES REGARDING HEALTH INSUR-
ANCE REIMBURSEMENT, PAYMENT, OR COPAYMENTS.

Cancellation Policy

STATE YOUR POLICY REGARDING CLIENT CANCELLATION AND
RESCHEDULING OF APPOINTMENTS.

Emergencies and Phone Consultations

DESCRIBE WHAT YOU WANT CLIENTS TO DO IN THE EVENT OF A MEN-
TAL-HEALTH EMERGENCY. STATE YOUR AVAILABILITY OR NONAVAIL-
ABILITY FOR EMERGENCIES AND PHONE CONSULTATIONS WITH
CLIENTS.

Coverage while Practitioner Is Unavailable

DESCRIBE WHAT YOU WANT CLIENTS TO DO IF THEY WANT TO REACH
YOU, AND YOU ARE OUT OF TOWN, ILL, OR OTHERWISE UNAVAIL-
ABLE. STATE HOW YOU ARRANGE FOR ANY BACKUP COVERAGE FOR
YOUR PRACTICE AND ANY ASSOCIATED POLICIES THAT YOU FOLLOW.

Grievances or Complaints

STATE YOUR POLICIES REGARDING THE RESOLUTION OF GRIEVANCES
OR COMPLAINTS BY CLIENTS AGAINST YOUR PRACTICE.

Signed Statement of Understanding and Consent

The Client's signature below indicates that he/she has read, understands, and
accepts this agreement and enters into it freely. If any part of this contract is
found to be invalid by a court of law or arbitration board, all other sections still
apply and are valid. The Client has received a copy of this document.

_____

Client Signature   Date

_____

NAME OF YOUR PRACTICE Representative   Date

Appendix D

Sample WHY Program Brochure

For Prospective Clients

NAME OF YOUR PRACTICE
ADDRESS
PHONE NUMBER
E-MAIL AND WEB SITE ADDRESSES

Achieve the Weight You Choose with Hypnosis!

The Weight, Hypnotherapy and YOU (WHY) Weight Reduction Program puts YOU IN CONTROL!

- Get Control Over What You Eat!
- Get Control Over How You Eat!
- Get Control Over Emotional Eating!
- Get Control Over Your Motivation to Exercise!
- Get Control Over Your Mind With the Power of Self-Hypnosis!

What You Receive in the Program Package:

- Eight sessions with NAME OF PRACTITIONER
- LIST SPECIAL TAKE-HOME MATERIALS, BOOKS, TAPES, OR MEDIA YOU CHOOSE TO INCLUDE IN THE PROGRAM
- Personalized weight reduction recordings, each 20–40 minutes in length
- WHY Program Client Handouts.

This program puts the control into your hands and enhances the choices you make about food and exercise. The hypnotic recordings reinforce your progress and allow you to design your own hypnotic suggestions! Incentives to succeed are built into the structure of the program, because you do not advance to the next step until you are successfully reducing your weight and shedding those excess pounds! Once you have achieved a reduction of at least SIXTEEN pounds, you have all the tools and methods you need to continue the program on your own, or, if you prefer, schedule additional sessions.

Note: To participate in this program, you must be under a medically supervised or physician-approved dietary/nutrition plan combined with a suitable exercise regimen.

The Eight Sessions

Session 1: Interview and Introduction

Session 2: Reframing Compulsive Eating

Session 3: Training in Self-Hypnosis

Session 4: Stopping Emotional Eating with Stress Management

After session 4, you will schedule each subsequent session when you have reduced your weight by at least four pounds. Once you reduce your weight by four pounds, schedule the next session right away. You are in charge, so you work at your own pace. You don't advance to the next step until you are ready and are actually losing weight.

For each of the following sessions you'll receive a customized recording of the hypnotherapy portion of that session. Listen to the recording as often as you wish to reinforce and enhance your progress.

Session 5: Making Sensible Food Choices

Session 6: Creating an Intelligent Relationship with Food

Session 7: Boosting Motivation to Exercise

Session 8: Pulling It All Together for Lasting Results

Price

STATE YOUR FEES AND PRICING STRUCTURE FOR THE PROGRAM.

Credentials and Biographical Sketch

LIST YOUR CREDENTIALS, PROFESSIONAL EXPERIENCE, AND AFFILIATIONS IN A BIOGRAPHICAL SKETCH.

Bonus Coupon

FOR CLIENTS WHO COMPLETE THE PROGRAM, INCLUDE A "BONUS COUPON" THAT OFFERS A "REFRESHER" OR FOLLOW-UP SESSION AT A DISCOUNTED FEE.

Other Information

HERE, INCLUDE CLIENT TESTIMONIALS, DIRECTIONS TO YOUR OFFICE, AND/OR OTHER SERVICES THAT YOU OFFER.

Sample WHY Weight Reduction Program Follow-up Letter

To follow up with clients who have completed the WHY Weight Reduction Program successfully, send a letter similar to the following on your letterhead.

Dear _____,

I am writing this letter to wish you continued success and satisfying results in weight reduction and maintenance. It has been my distinct pleasure to help you toward reaching your target weight.

Let this letter serve as a reminder to continue proper medical care, nutrition, and exercise. Continue to listen to the recordings that accompany the Weight, Hypnotherapy and YOU Weight Reduction Program to reinforce your progress. Feel free to call me regarding any questions or concerns about the program or about my services.

I also invite you to consider additional sessions on issues related to personal health, body image, and weight maintenance. I offer sessions on self-esteem, relaxation, stress management, confidence building, making effective life transitions, assertive communication skills, conflict resolution, and finding your life purpose.

If you are happy with the results of the work we've done together, please tell your friends. I've enclosed an extra WHY Program brochure for you to pass along to someone else who might benefit from my services.

I wish you all the rewards of good health!

YOUR SIGNATURE

Appendix F

Eighteen Ways to Induce and Deepen Hypnotic Trance

"You are going deeper ... deeper." How many times a day does a hypnotherapist say these words? Would you like to add some variety to your deepening methods? Here are eighteen things you can say to induce and deepen hypnotic trance. Each item on the list has a short script as an example. You will recognize several hypnotic language patterns. Keep in mind that some methods overlap. Read all the scripts in the entire list sequentially, and you will have an effective trance induction for relaxation.

Begin by encouraging the client to get comfortable. You may want to give the client the choice of closing the eyes; staring at some object, such as a candle flame; or just looking at a blank wall.

1. Ask the client to take a deep breath and relax

   Ease back and take a deep breath, all the way in. As you slowly let it out, perhaps you can feel your muscles beginning to relax, at the same time that your mind is just beginning to pay attention in a different way.

2. Pace the client's current experience with truisms and lead into trance.

   You are listening to my voice and the sounds in the room. You are aware of your surroundings. You are aware of the position of your arms and legs. You can feel the texture of your clothing. You can feel the support of the chair on which you are sitting. You notice your breathing, and you notice how much more relaxed and calm you feel now than you did just moments ago.

3. Reassure the client that trance is easy to attain and he or she is a good candidate for hypnosis.

   Going into trance is different for each person, and whatever way you experience it is just fine. I am sure you can do this.

4. Compounding:

   The more you listen, the more you relax. The more you relax, the easier it is to go within and achieve that level of inner awareness where special learning takes place.

5.   Fractionation:

As you learn to go into trance, you can practice for improvement. Open your eyes for a moment. Look around. Now close your eyes and go right back to an even more satisfying level of relaxation and concentration. [Repeat two or three times.]

6.   Imply cause-and-effect:

As you wonder what hypnosis is all about, you understand more. Each breath you exhale can make it more satisfying. Each moment that passes brings you a greater sense of comfort. With each breath, you can advance more completely into relaxation and concentration.

7.   Suggest many possibilities:

People go into trance in a wide variety of ways, and everyone's experience is unique. Some people relax quickly, some relax more slowly, and some vary the pace. Some people hear every word I say, but others tune my voice in and out. Or you might devote your attention to your own thoughts and not really listen at all. For some, trance is a light, floating experience; for others it is a deep, heavy experience; and for some, it is a combination of sensations. How you create this experience for yourself is really up to you—you can just relax and discover what happens naturally. It may be what you expect, or something you don't expect, or some of both.

8.   Eye closure:

Now relax your eyelids and all the muscles around your eyes even more than before. Let your eyelids feel heavy and drowsy. Let your eyelids relax so much that they just don't feel like opening. They feel so heavy, so relaxed that if you tried to open them, you'd find it difficult. Now relax your eyelids so much more that they just want to stay shut. Later on, of course, they will open easily, but for now you can enjoy the feeling of allowing your subconscious to take part in this process, relaxing your eyelids so much they just stay closed. Now test your eyelids to be sure they want to stay shut. Very good! Now stop testing and experience the satisfaction of realizing that your mind and body are fully cooperating with the process of hypnosis, as you relax more peacefully.

9.   Progressive relaxation: suggest that each part of the body is relaxing. Be sure to pause between each sentence, giving the client time to respond.

Send the thought of relaxation all the way down to your feet and feel your feet relaxing. Allow the same relaxation to move gently upward through your body, into your ankles and calves. Let the relaxing sensations continue, so that now your knees and thighs feel more relaxed, as the relaxation moves into your hips and abdomen. Now feel the muscles of your back beginning to relax. Even your shoulders relax, as comforting sensations flow down into your chest and each breath you exhale helps deepen that sense of relaxation and letting go. Let the relaxation flow down your arms, into your elbows, down into your wrists, and all the way down to the tips of your fingers. Your entire body is relaxing more, while that soothing feeling moves into your neck and your scalp, and all the muscles of your face relax. Your entire body feels relaxed from head to toe.

10. **Presuppose that deepening is occurring:**

    I wonder how completely you are relaxing. You are discovering for yourself how satisfying trance can be. While you are relaxing, many subtle changes are occurring.

11. **Describe some common aspects of trance:**

    Your breathing might be slower and more regular. Perhaps your muscles are more relaxed, and your hands might feel loose and limp, while your heartbeat and pulse are slowing down. You may be finding it easier to concentrate on the things I say, although from time to time, you are thinking your own thoughts, too.

12. **Splitting: Pose to the client that he or she is aware of two opposite things at once. Use a different tone of voice for each one.**

    You have a conscious mind … *and you have a subconscious mind.* Your conscious mind is aware of the external world … *and your subconscious mind manages your inner awareness.* The conscious mind deals with facts and logic … *while the subconscious mind works with intuition and creativity.* The conscious mind thinks about the problems … *while the subconscious mind holds the solutions.* Mere conversation speaks to the conscious mind … *and hypnosis speaks to the subconscious mind.*

13. **Revivify a memory of previous trance (if it was pleasant) or a similar experience of comfort and relaxation. Note: Ask the client to describe the previous experience before you begin hypnosis. Then use the client's own words here, as you help the client access the memory.**

    I'm sure you can remember that previous time when you experienced hypnosis. You might recall some of your thoughts and observations and the sensations you felt as your body relaxed and your mind seemed to "focus inward," as though you were "drifting effortlessly" while feeling comfortable and secure. You remember that it was "a soothing feeling to let go of all that stress." You can have the same satisfying feelings now.

14. **Metaphor or analogy:**

    Some people say going into trance is as comfortable as going to bed at night, at the end of a long, productive day, with nothing left to do but close your eyes and let go and relax. There are no distractions and nothing to think about. You can just let your mind drift, feeling warm and comfortable, while enjoying the peace and quiet.

15. **Counting:**

    I am going to count now from 1 to 5. With each number, just let your mind and body relax more and more, so that by the time I reach the number 5, you will be much more deeply relaxed, with a fuller sense of inner awareness. One, relaxing deeper and deeper. Two, relaxing more and completely. Three, a deeply comfortable feeling. Four, going within to find what is there to discover. Five, much more relaxed now.

16. Guided imagery:

Imagine you are drifting down a quiet stream in a canoe, under a lovely blue sky. The current carries you along, so you can just sit back and relax and enjoy the scenery. Overhead, an occasional cloud floats slowly by, moving effortlessly with its own sense of direction, even though you don't know where it is going. It changes shape as it moves, sometimes resembling something recognizable, sometimes not. On either side of you, you see the riverbank, with trees, grasses, shrubs, and flowers. Butterflies flit among the colorful flowers, seeming to know just what to do to get at that sweet nectar deep inside each one. All is peaceful and tranquil, as you let the current carry you, and the gentle rocking of the canoe, under the warmth of the sun, is lulling you into a deeply restful state.

17. Arm catalepsy:

As you focus inward, you can notice how relaxed your arms are. Let them feel so relaxed that they feel rested, so comfortable. It's as though they just don't want to move. They are so heavy and relaxed, it's just too much effort to move them. Try to lift your right arm and find that you'd rather not lift it, or that it is so heavy, it just doesn't want to lift. Stop trying and relax even more comfortably. This should give you an indication that you are now fully in hypnotic trance, and how pleasant and peaceful it can be for you.

18. Word play:

As you trance-ition into hypnotic trance in your own way, getting out of your own way, you might trance-fer some previous learning to have it your own way, or it could be that you wait for the experience to trance-form your awareness of how you own the way you do it and trance-late what I say, into something you can use now or later, or have discovered earlier on.

This piece was adapted from an article by Judith E. Pearson, originally published in Interlink, *the newsletter of the National Board for Certified Clinical Hypnotherapists, Silver Spring, Maryland, 1997.*

Appendix G

Introduction to Clinical Hypnosis and Hypnotherapy

Judith E. Pearson, Ph.D.

What Are Hypnosis and Trance?

Hypnosis is a method of communication that induces a trance. Hypnosis can be conducted by one individual addressing another, or it may be conducted by the self addressing the subconscious (self-hypnosis). Trance is a naturally occurring state in which one's attention is narrowly focused and relatively free of distractions. People go into and out of trance spontaneously throughout the day, mostly when concentrating on something. In trance, the attention may be focused either internally (on thoughts—through internal self-talk, images, or both) or externally (on a task, a book, or a movie, for example). The focus of attention is so narrow that other stimuli in the environment are ignored or blocked out of conscious awareness for a time. Examples of trance states are daydreaming, deep concentration, and some forms of meditation.

Clinical hypnosis was approved by the American Medical Association in 1958. Clinical hypnosis, also called *hypnotherapy*, is the use of hypnosis in a medical, psycho-educational, or therapeutic setting. Hypnotherapy is rarely used in isolation. It is one of many therapeutic methods available to a practitioner. A skilled practitioner will combine clinical hypnosis with other methods such as cognitive therapy, client-centered therapy, psychodynamics, eye-movement therapy, thought field therapy, Neuro-Linguistic Programming, and other brief, solution-oriented approaches. Clinical hypnosis is best suited to individual counseling and is generally not recommended for couples counseling, marriage and family therapy, or group counseling.

As an adjunct to psychotherapy or counseling, clinical hypnosis can help the client obtain a relaxed, comfortable, trance state for visualizing and obtaining specific therapeutic outcomes. It is theorized that trance increases suggestibility. With clinical hypnosis, the therapist can make suggestions designed to help the client formulate specific internal processes (feelings, memories, images, and self-talk) that can lead to mutually agreed-upon outcomes—changes in behavior and emotions. Hypnotic suggestions can best influence subsequent behavior when the listener is (a) cooperative, relaxed, receptive, and open to the suggestions; (b) motivated to get the outcome; and (c) anticipates and envisions that the suggestions will result in success.

Formal trance methods usually include instructions for relaxation and concentration. Trance is facilitated through *hypnotic language patterns,* which include guided visualization; stories; accessing memories; analogies; ambiguous words or phrases; repetition; and statements about association, meaning, and cause-and-effect. A hypnotherapist may make references to those aspects of the mind that are not readily available to conscious awareness. This part of the mind may be variously referred to as the subconscious mind, the unconscious mind, the inner mind, a "part" of your mind, or your higher wisdom.

Myths and Misconceptions about Clinical Hypnosis

Hypnosis is not mind control or brainwashing. Research has shown that attempts to "brainwash" people through extreme methods such as physical and mental duress have proven ineffective, except in causing states of depression, anxiety, and confusion. Some people worry that hypnosis could cause them to do something against their will or that could endanger them. Research shows that this is not the case. Hypnosis is a method of influence, and, depending on the skills of the practitioner and the receptivity of the listener, it is no more or less powerful than any other kind or method of psychological persuasion, manipulation, or motivation (such as advertising or propaganda). The difference is that a qualified clinical hypnotherapist is guided by legal requirements and ethical responsibilities. Therefore, the therapist is required to work contractually with the client toward specific outcomes, under informed consent and with mutual agreement. In the clinical environment, rapport, trust, and cooperation are essential for the success of hypnotherapy—or, in fact, for any other kind of psychotherapy.

People change their minds and actions throughout their lives. When such changes occur as a result of exposure to specific information, it is sometimes because this information has been presented through skillful persuasion and influence. A hypnotherapist uses communicative methods of persuasion and influence; so do people who advertise and market goods and services; so do teachers, politicians, lawyers, entertainers, parents, and ministers.

During light trance, you are not immobilized. You remain aware of your surroundings. In light trance, people can open their eyes, talk, and move around. In fact, most people in this stage of trance are not aware of being "hypnotized." Most people can be hypnotized to some degree. Anyone who can be hypnotized can also be easily taught to bring himself or herself out of trance at any time. In fact, emerging from trance happens spontaneously when one is interrupted, as by a phone ringing.

The deepest levels of trance produce a dreamlike state. Some people become so relaxed in trance that they may fall asleep. This is not a problem because some part of the mind continues to listen to the voice of the hypnotherapist. Under hypnosis, many sleeping clients can still follow instructions such as moving a finger, taking a deep breath, or awakening themselves when told to do so. Many people require practice and training to routinely reach deep trance states, while a few people seem to have a natural ability to do so.

There is no "right" way to experience trance. People vary in suggestibility depending on their personality traits and moods. Some people enter trance easily, and some don't. One person may find it a deep, restful feeling, while another may experience a light, floating sensation. Some people hear every word the hypnotherapist says, while others allow their minds to drift to other thoughts. Some experience vivid imagery, while others do not. Some people remember the suggestions they hear, and some do not. Some people see results right away, and some people see results gradually over time, or even after a delay of a few days or weeks. Every person's experience of hypnosis is unique.

Additionally, there are dozens of ways to induce trance and make hypnotic suggestions. If one way doesn't work well for you, or doesn't seem to produce results, don't give up. Give your therapist some feedback on what is and isn't working, so that he or she can choose another method.

Hypnosis cannot solve every problem. Even with hypnosis, it is still necessary for you to do some conscientious planning and research about the outcome you choose. You should still expect to make conscious decisions, and you will have to take action to get results. Hypnosis is not a cure-all and it is not magic. Hypnosis can be effective in many cases, but there are no guarantees that hypnosis will work for everyone under every circumstance.

Risks and Precautions

Hypnosis carries very few risks. It is contraindicated for individuals with certain medical problems, for those who are actively abusing drugs or alcohol, or for those who are paranoid, psychotic, delusional, or hallucinatory. Hypnosis should not be used for physical problems, such as pain, unless the client has first consulted a physician to determine the underlying physical causes.

Formal hypnotic methods are not recommended for small children, because children lack the necessary attention span. More interactive treatment methods can be used, however, such as art therapy, play therapy, storytelling, and guided visualization, during which helpful suggestions can be made to the child.

Some clients request hypnotherapy for the purpose of recovering memories. Hypnosis may or may not be effective in this regard. Human memory is subjective, illusive, and sometimes distorted. There is no reliable way to "make" someone remember what he or she has forgotten, although hypnosis sometimes helps. When memories do surface in therapy, there is no guarantee that they are accurate or based on reality. False memories can occur not just under hypnosis, but in other circumstances as well.

In rare cases, after trance work, the person may feel somewhat disoriented. The therapist should ensure that you are fully alert and sufficiently energized to leave the therapist's office and continue the day's activities safely. In very rare cases, after a hypnotic session some people may experience mildly disturbing thoughts or feelings. If this happens, you should call your therapist immediately for a follow-up session.

Ericksonian Hypnosis

The type of hypnotherapy most frequently practiced today is *Ericksonian hypnosis,* named after the late Milton H. Erickson, M.D. From the 1930s to the 1980s Erickson was highly influential in integrating clinical hypnosis with medicine and psychotherapy. His hypnotic methods were permissive and respectful of the client. He established the American Society for Clinical Hypnosis and published the first professional journals and monographs on therapeutic hypnosis. The Ericksonian Foundation continues his work. Numerous books and articles have been written about Erickson and his methods. Mental-health practitioners and clinicians can obtain training in Ericksonian hypnosis through continuing education and postgraduate programs. Certified hypnotherapists are those who have met the credentialing standards of a national board or credentialing organization.

Appendix H

What Is Neuro-Linguistic Programming?

By Judith E. Pearson, Ph.D.

Neuro-Linguistic Programming (NLP) is a cutting-edge branch of psychology with applications for coaching, psychotherapy, sports, business, sales, and behavioral health. It can be combined with and used to enhance methods of teaching and communication. This article will explain the history of NLP, what it is, and what it can do for *you*.

Background

In the 1970s, two researchers at the University of Santa Cruz, in California—Richard Bandler and Dr. John Grinder—conducted a linguistic study of the leading psychotherapists of the day. Bandler and Grinder analyzed the communication patterns of Virginia Satir (a renowned family therapist), Dr. Fritz Perls (founder of gestalt psychotherapy), and Dr. Milton Erickson (psychiatrist and internationally famous hypnotherapist). Drawing from Alfred Korzybski's work in general semantics, Bandler and Grinder modeled the language patterns of these psychotherapists and distilled a method of psychotherapy called NLP.

They taught others how to use NLP to facilitate lasting, dramatic behavioral change in a short time. Certified NLP practitioners and trainers formed training institutes across the United States and Europe. In the 1980s, practitioners took NLP into sports, health, business, and sales training, teaching people to achieve excellence. Today, NLP is practiced and taught worldwide, with hundreds of books and workshop offerings on the subject.

NLP Philosophy

NLP is based on some basic philosophical tenets about human nature. These ideas aren't necessarily universal truths, but rather are useful ways of thinking about people and self-improvement. Here are a few:

- People do not operate on reality. They operate on their internal maps of reality. These maps are always imperfect. NLP helps us understand our maps and improve them.

- People perceive the world through their senses. People's thoughts and emotions are internal images, conversations and sounds, physical sensations, and remembered tastes and smells. In NLP we call these internal channels *visual, auditory, kinesthetic, and olfactory/gustatory.* By describing internal processes in these terms, we can describe to others our internal ways of thinking and feeling.

- Human thoughts, behaviors, and feelings have structures, or patterns. NLP improves those structures, so that people have increased flexibility in their thinking, behavior, and feelings.

- Self-improvement methods are not useful, lasting, or effective if they conflict with a person's core needs and values. NLP teaches people to honor their needs and values in order to feel congruent about the changes they make.

- The causes of some behaviors and emotions lie outside conscious awareness. NLP works with both the conscious mind and the "subconscious" mind, through hypnotic processes.

- People communicate both verbally and nonverbally. NLP helps people to better understand the meaning of both kinds of communication.

- People have the internal resources they need to make the changes they desire. NLP helps people access these resources.

- Most behaviors, even problematic ones, are based on underlying positive intentions, which may reside in the unconscious mind. NLP brings about the insights that explain these underlying motivations.

NLP Methods

NLP is based on communication patterns and structured cognitive exercises that combine conversation, hypnotic language, trance work, metaphor, visualization, eye movements, physical movement, breathing, and posture. NLP is process oriented.

NLP helps people change their behavioral-cognitive-emotional "states" so that they can alter their behaviors. Typically, an NLP session begins with a client identifying and describing a specific aspect of behavior he or she wishes to improve or change. The NLP practitioner will ask questions designed to help define the problem. The client then describes the "outcome," or "solution," to the problem. Then the NLP practitioner guides the client through a step-by-step process to obtain the solution. A single NLP process can take from ten minutes to two hours, and most practitioners work in forty-five- to sixty-minute sessions. NLP methods work for individuals, groups, children, and adults. NLP methods are gentle and respectful of the individual.

Generally, NLP processes teach people to

- understand and communicate their thought processes more coherently
- see problems from a new perspective
- steer their thinking in a new direction
- access personal strengths and inner resources
- focus on the solution, rather than on the problem
- focus on what can be done, rather than on why something happened
- heal traumatic events of the past
- feel empowered to cope with difficulties more effectively
- think optimistically about future possibilities
- gain insight into the unconscious sources of some behaviors
- feel congruent about the changes they make in their lives
- expand their behavioral choices, to allow greater adaptation and flexibility.

Appendix I

The NLP Slender Eating Strategy

This strategy will help you develop a healthy relationship with food, eat sensibly, and curb a tendency to eat because of emotions or external triggers. This adaptation of the NLP Naturally Slender Eating Strategy is a way to make decisions about food, eating, and hunger in the same way a Trim-Slim person would—except that a Trim-Slim person does so automatically, without conscious thought. The procedure was originally developed by NLP trainers Connirae and Steve Andreas and is described in their book *Heart of the Mind*.

Instructions: Apply this variation of the NLP Naturally Slender Eating Strategy at least once a day for the next week. You can use it during a snack or an entire meal.

Step 1

When you feel the urge to eat something, stop whatever you are doing at the moment. Sit down and get quiet with yourself. Concentrate on your inner responses. Ask yourself what is prompting you to eat at this moment.

- Is it some cue in your environment, such as the sight or smell of food, the time of day, or talk about food?
- Is it some emotion, such as boredom, anger, anxiety, worry, fear, guilt, loneliness, or disappointment?
- Is it because you don't like yourself right now, or don't like your life right now?
- Is it that you feel happy and you are celebrating something; or perhaps you want to reward yourself?
- Or is it that you truly feel hungry: your stomach is empty, and your body needs an energy boost?

If your answer falls in one of the first four categories, be aware that your desire to eat is due not to hunger, but to something else. You now have a choice. Decide if you really want food, or if there is something else you want. You are learning to distinguish hunger from other eating triggers. If you decide you aren't really hungry, and you choose to do something other than eat, you can stop the process here. Otherwise, if you really are hungry, or you really do need an energy boost, go on to step 2.

Step 2

If you've decided to eat something, this step will help you decide what to eat. Concentrate on the sensations in your mouth and stomach. In the beginning you might find it helpful to close your eyes for this step and to place the palm of your hand on your stomach area, just below your rib cage. Ask yourself, "What would taste good in my mouth and feel good in my stomach right now?" Think over the foods that are available to you and acceptable to you. You might be thinking about what you have on hand in the kitchen if you are at home, or about what is on the menu if you are in a restaurant.

Step 3

Think of a food (or combination of foods) you could eat. Now imagine eating a serving of that food. Think about how the food will taste and feel in your mouth, how it will feel as you swallow it. Does it seem that this food (or food combination) will be satisfying, in terms of smell, taste, and texture? If not, think of another possibility. Test out the options in your mind until you find an acceptable food that will satisfy your mouth.

Step 4

Now think about how much of this food (or combination of foods) you want to eat. Again, place your hand on your stomach, close your eyes, and ask yourself, "How much of this food will give me a satisfied feeling of fullness in my stomach? Do I want just a small portion to fill a small space, a medium-sized portion to fill a medium space, or a full meal to fill my whole stomach?" Sometimes you can get an intuitive indication, before eating, of just how much you want to eat. Remember, the average adult human stomach can comfortably hold only about two heaping handfuls of food—that should give you a starting point. If this step doesn't work for you, don't worry. Just take a small portion for now and go on to the next step.

Step 5

Think about how you will feel immediately after you have eaten this food in this amount. Think about how you will feel an hour afterward. Will you feel satisfied? Will you feel guilty? Will you wish you had eaten something else? If you anticipate feeling guilt or regret, maybe your food choice isn't the best you could make. Go back to step 2 and start again. Consider other choices. When you have a choice that will leave you satisfied, without guilt or regret, then go on to step 6.

Step 6

Now begin to eat slowly and attentively, concentrating your attention on each bite. It's ideal to do this exercise alone. If you are with a companion and want to have a conversation, however, just put your fork down between bites, while you talk. Taking a drink of water between bites is another way to eat more slowly.

While you are eating, pause every few bites, put down your fork, and breathe deeply. At each pause, focus your attention on the feeling in your stomach. Again, you might want to place the palm of your hand on your stomach, pressing in gently. Notice the difference in the way your stomach feels now, with food in it, compared to how it did when you first began this exercise, with no or little food in your stomach. Remain aware of the feeling in your stomach as you continue to eat slowly. It might even help to picture the amount of food you have eaten, as it begins to take up the space in your stomach. Continue eating until you are aware of that comfortable, not-quite-full feeling. Now pause for a minute to notice whether that not-quite-full feeling develops into a comfortably full feeling in your stomach. If not, take another bite and wait a minute. Keep taking one bite at a time until you get that satisfied, full feeling. You might notice other changes, too—perhaps a sense of contentment or more mental alertness, depending on what you've eaten.

Step 7

When you are aware of that full feeling, stop eating. Put your fork down and push your plate away. It doesn't matter if there is food left on it or if someone offers you a second helping. It doesn't matter if someone else encourages you to eat more. Just say, "No thanks. I've eaten enough and I don't want any more. I'm not hungry now." Get up and leave the table or, if you are in a restaurant, ask the wait staff to remove your plate.

Feel a sense of accomplishment that you are learning to eat according to your body's communications. Soon you will develop the habit of eating healthful foods when you feel hungry, in just the right amount to satisfy your hunger, and you'll stop eating when you feel full.

When You've Completed This Exercise

When you've practiced this exercise once a day for a week, think about everything you learned and answer the following questions.

- What steps of the process worked for you?

- For the steps of the process that worked for you, how did they help?
- Is there some way you could modify this process to better meet your needs?
- What improvements in your eating habits did you notice over the course of the week?

Now envision that over the next few days and weeks you are applying what you learned from this assignment as you enhance your relationship with food, and you find that you are making progress toward your preferred weight.

The NLP Slender Eating Strategy was developed by NLP trainers and practitioners Connirae and Steve Andreas and is described in their book: Heart of the Mind *(Moab, UT: Real People Press, 1989).*

Appendix J

Report: The Benefits of Exercise

If all the benefits of exercise could be squeezed into a pill, it would be considered a miracle drug—the "rejuvenation pill." Everyone would want it and would be willing to pay thousands of dollars for the extraordinary advantages—which come with no side-effects! No one would want to be without it. So why don't more people get off their behinds and exercise?

Newspapers, books, television shows, and magazines extol the benefits of physical exercise and activity as a means to physical fitness and a longer life. In every town and city in the United States you can find bike paths, jogging trails, health clubs, gyms, racquet clubs, tennis courts, aerobics classes, dance studios, martial arts classes, and community recreation facilities. You would surmise that the country is caught up in a frenzy of fitness. Although it is true that our population values exercise more than ever before, it is also true that obesity has reached epidemic proportions in this land of abundance and affluence. One-third of the population is overweight. In Black and Hispanic cultures and in low-income groups, 50 percent of the women are obese. Life doesn't have to be that way—and you don't have to be in the "fat people" category.

Regular exercise brings more than an improved physique. Exercise can help you *sleep better, manage stress more effectively, strengthen your heart, prevent osteoporosis, burn calories, decrease your appetite, improve your skin, and bolster your self-esteem*—and even more! WOW! Physical activity, combined with good nutrition, can actually slow the aging process itself. Let's look more closely at the rewards of exercise.

Exercise conditions your body to function more efficiently. The physical benefits of exercise are:

Improved circulation, a stronger heart, and improved lung capacity: Aerobic activity works the heart muscle, increases blood flow, and makes the lungs pump harder—strengthening the entire cardiovascular system.

Healthier skin: Exercise increases circulation, bringing blood flow to the skin surface, carrying nutrients and flushing away toxins. Your skin looks younger, has a glow, and is healthier.

Prevention of osteoporosis: Weight-bearing exercises, such as walking, strengthen bones and slow down bone loss due to aging.

Increased metabolism: Exercise burns calories and keeps the metabolic rate high for hours, even after the activity has ended.

Increased muscle tone: If you are dieting and reducing your food intake without exercising, you are losing muscle instead of fat. Muscle burns many more calories than fat, by a ratio of thirty to one. In order to retain muscle, you must exercise. Muscle weighs more than fat, but the tissue is denser and takes up less space, so you look slimmer as you build muscle tissues and burn more calories stored in fat.

Rehabilitation from muscular-skeletal injuries: Under the supervision of a sports physician or physical therapist, targeted exercises and movement can facilitate repair of damaged muscles, ligaments, and tendons. Sometimes even old injuries can improve with the proper exercise.

Exercise also gives you these psychological benefits:

Relief from stress and mild, transitory depression: Studies show that people who exercise have less stress. Exercise is a healthy way to work off frustration and anger. It gives "time out" from the demands of work and family. Increased circulation pumps oxygen to the brain for clearer thinking. Activities involving the whole body activate neurological activity across both hemispheres of the brain, which can have a calming effect.

Regulation of brain chemistry: A study by Nora Volkow, reported in the November–December 2004 issue of *Psychology Today* (McGowan 2004), found that the brains of obese people were deficient in dopamine—a chemical involved in motivation, pleasure, and learning. The deficiency creates a "craving for stimulation" that prompts overeating and other addictions. As the addictive response develops over time, the prefrontal cortex, the part of the brain associated with judgment and inhibition, stops functioning normally. The antidote is prolonged, regular exercise, which causes the brain to release endorphins and elevates dopamine levels. Endorphins are the brain's own "feel good" chemicals (the release of endorphins causes the "runner's high" experienced by distance runners).

Increased self-esteem: Meeting a physical challenge—like finishing a ten-kilometer race or hiking a mountain trail or swimming twenty laps in a pool—brings the exhilaration of accomplishment and an enhanced sense of competence and mastery. Some people enjoy the camaraderie and fellowship of team sports and the shared fun of group activity. Some enjoy the improved grace that comes from activities involving precision movement like dance, swimming, or gymnastics. Exercise can enhance your sense of self-worth.

There is no pill, no medical treatment, no cosmetic preparation that can equal the benefits of regular physical exercise. Given these fantastic benefits, you can't pass it up! Exercise is absolutely essential to your health and well-being!

How to Get Started on an Exercise Routine

If you are not yet into an exercise routine, here are some ways to get started on a sensible regimen that will transform your mind, body, and spirit! The key to success is to set reasonable, incremental goals for yourself, so that you build strength and stamina slowly and safely over time. Follow these guidelines to developing an exercise routine:

Consult with your physician first: Get a complete physical exam and ask your physician about the types of exercise that are safe for you.

Choose a mix of activities: Ideally, you want an exercise routine that includes stretching exercises for flexibility, aerobic activity for cardiovascular fitness, and resistance exercises for strength and toning.

Consider a trainer: For optimal results, consult with a personal trainer who can help you design an exercise routine based on your age, physical condition, and fitness goals. A trainer is especially important if you plan to use weights or exercise machines. A personal trainer can help you start out at the proper speed and level of resistance, show you the proper postures and movements, and teach you how to avoid injury.

Get the right gear: Make sure you are wearing the proper clothing for your activity—that might mean footwear, protective knee pads, gloves, helmet, or a jogging bra or athletic supporter. If you use equipment, it should be in excellent condition and well maintained.

Warm up and stretch: At the beginning of your routine, spend about five minutes warming up—for example, walking in place or freestyle dancing—to get the blood circulating to your muscles and to loosen up your joints. Then stretch slowly until you feel some resistance and hold each stretch for a count of ten to twenty seconds. Warming up helps avoid muscle sprains.

Start slowly and pay attention to your body's responses: During the first days and weeks of a new exercise routine, be careful and don't push too hard. Limit your initial workouts to a few minutes of light activity—or to a few minutes more than you usually do. If you feel fatigue or pain, stop and rest and try again tomorrow. Build strength and stamina over several weeks or months, and increase the demands on your body gradually.

Make it fun: Do exercise you enjoy. Exercise alone in the privacy of your home or with a friend or go to a gym or join a class. If you think your routine is getting dull, build in some variety. Exercise to music, walk with your pooch, bicycle with your child, watch TV while you work out, take dance lessons with your spouse—the list is endless.

Chart your progress: Put a chart on your refrigerator that shows how many sit-ups you do each day or how many miles you walk or how many minutes you spend on the treadmill. Or just put a big gold star on the calendar for every day you exercise. Soon you will like what you see!

Integrate movement into your daily routine: You'll get more from exercise (and burn additional calories) if you move around and stay active during the day. If you sit most of the day, take breaks at least every hour and stand up, stretch, take a few deep breaths, and walk around for a few minutes.

Make an appointment with yourself for exercise time, and give that time top priority. Keep the appointment, as if it were an appointment to receive a million dollars or meet with world leaders or interview for your dream job or go on a date with someone you adore. Get into a daily routine, so you actually begin to look forward to exercising. Don't miss it for anything except an emergency. Don't let others talk you out of it. Make exercise time sacred and non-negotiable. Exercise is for you, to make you feel good and look good, and you are worth it!

Portions of this report were excerpted and adapted from Healthy Habits: Total Conditioning for a Healthy Body and Mind, *by Kathy Corsetty and Judith E. Pearson (Lincoln, NE: Dageforde Press, 2000).*

Appendix K

Report: Brain-Health Recommendations to Curb Compulsive Eating

According to neuropsychiatrist Daniel Amen, compulsive eating and binging may sometimes be symptoms of depression, fatigue, imbalance in blood sugars, chemical imbalances in the brain, such as reduced serotonin levels, or some combination of these factors. Amen (Amen & Routh 2004) has recently published several books on the interactions between brain chemistry and lifestyle. He writes that depression, compulsions, and anxiety are sometimes the outward indications of brain-activity dysfunctions caused by any number of factors, including exposure to toxic substances, genetics, stress, trauma, high fevers, head injury, or a poor diet—even though some of these risk factors may have occurred much earlier in the person's life. If you suspect your client's compulsive eating may be associated with a brain chemistry malfunction, you may choose to recommend a complete neurological examination. You might also want to share with your client the brain-health recommendations (which are also contained in a handout in the *Client Workbook*).[12]

- Get a complete physical exam. Ideally, the exam should include tests for blood sugar, lipids and cholesterol levels (via blood sampling), and brain-activity patterns (via brain imaging).

- Take a daily multivitamin containing B complex vitamins at the dosage recommended on the label.

- Take 1,000 milligrams of fish oil or omega-3 fatty acids daily.

- Eliminate alcohol, nicotine, and illegal drugs. All these substances have the potential to damage the brain and may aggravate existing brain problems and emotional difficulties.

- Limit exposure to toxic chemicals, such as spray paints, insecticides, and so on.

- Studies show conclusively that inadequate sleep affects hormones associated with mood and appetite, and correlates with weight gain. Get eight hours of uninterrupted sleep each night. Avoid caffeine and stimulating activity late in the day. Drink milk (providing you are not lactose intolerant or allergic to dairy products) or take melatonin (75 milligrams orally) at bedtime. Resting in a dark, quiet room may help with falling asleep. Do not take melatonin in combination with supplements containing magnesium or zinc.

• Switch to a diet high in protein, eating five or six small portions throughout the day.

• Choose complex carbohydrates (vegetables, fresh fruits, and whole grains) over processed foods containing refined sugars and simple carbohydrates (white bread, baked goods, pasta, white rice, and potatoes). Consult a nutritionist as needed.

• Take Saint-John's-wort (for adults, 600 milligrams in the morning and 300 milligrams before bed). Saint-John's-wort is contraindicated for women who are taking birth-control pills or are pregnant or breast-feeding. When taking Saint-John's-wort, avoid foods and beverages containing tyramine, such as Chianti wine, beer, aged cheese, chicken livers, chocolate, bananas, and meat tenderizers. Avoid sun exposure. Caution: Saint-John's-wort may have adverse interactions with prescription antidepressants, lithium, alcohol, birth-control pills, cold and allergy drugs, flu medicines, decongestants, protease inhibitors for HIV, amphetamines, and narcotic pain relievers. Always consult a physician or pharmacist about the possible interactions between nutritional and herbal supplements and prescription or over-the-counter medications.

• L-tryptophan and 5-HTP are nutritional supplements that may boost serotonin levels in the brain. The recommended dosage for adults is 1,000 to 3,000 milligrams of L-tryptophan at bedtime and 50 to 100 milligrams of 5-HTP three times daily, with or without food. L-tryptophan may have an adverse interaction with antidepressants, lithium, and other prescription medications such as Imitrex and Ambien. Again, always consult a physician or pharmacist about the possible interactions between nutritional and herbal supplements and prescription or over-the-counter medications.

• Get adequate daily physical activity.

• Exposure to sunlight may also help, if you are not taking Saint-John's-wort. The brain seems to respond well to natural light. Sunlight activates vitamin D in the skin, which supports the brain's production of tryptophan—nature's own tranquilizer. Just use sunscreen to protect the skin from UV rays.

- If you have sleep problems or depression, consult a physician concerning the value and possible side-effects of prescription antidepressants and sleep-enhancing medications.

References

Amen, D. G., and L. C. Routh. 2004. *Healing Anxiety and Depression*. New York: Berkeley Books.

Gangwisch, J. et al. 2004. Lack of Sleep May Lead to Excess Weight. Paper presented to the North American Association for the Study of Obesity Annual Scientific Meeting, November 14–18, 2004, Las Vegas, Nevada. [Abstract 42-OR]

Mignot, E. et al. 2004. Stanford Study Links Obesity to Hormonal Changes from Lack of Sleep. *Public Library of Science*, Dec. 6. (Cited on Stanford University Medical Center, Office of Communication and Public Affairs web site.)

Taheri, S. 2004. The Mechanisms for the Interaction between Sleep and Metabolism. Available online at the University of Bristol, Laboratories for Integrative Neurosciences and Endocrinology web site <www.bris.ac.uk/neuroscience/research/research/groups/pidetails/105>.

Notes

1. Anthony Robbins is an internationally recognized motivational speaker, author, and trainer whose work is founded on the principles and methods of Neuro-Linguistic Programming.

2. Bariatrics is the branch of medicine dealing with the causes, prevention, and pharmacological and surgical treatment of obesity.

3. Ron Klein gave permission to relate this anecdote.

4. Sources: Health Survey for England with additional data from World Health Organization (1998), "Obesity: Preventing and Managing the Global Epidemic"; Expert Group Convened by Health Promotion Directorate (1988), "Canadian Guidelines for Healthy Weights"; and U.S. Department of Health and Human Services (2006), *How Is BMI Calculated and Interpreted?*

5. Source: American Cancer Society: "Calculate Your Daily Calorie Needs" (2006). These numbers may vary slightly according to the source one consults. Individual calorie needs may also vary from those recommended here.

6. Some parts of this induction were adapted from Morrill (2000).

7. Adapted from Allen 2004.

8. Adapted from Thompson in Kane and Olness 2004: Sand Bucket Induction.

9. Many of the ideas in this script were inspired and adapted from a transcript of Richard Bandler's work with an overweight demonstration subject in *The Spirit of NLP*, by L. Michael Hall (Bancyfelin, Wales: Anglo American Book Co., 1995). Used with permission of L. Michael Hall, Ph.D.

10. Adapted from Preston 2001.

11. Variations on this "healing light" visualization can be found in many texts. For this script I drew from Battino (2000).

12. These recommendations have been reviewed by a professional nutritionist. This report is not intended as a cure for any disease or substitute for medical advice. If symptoms are severe or persistent, consult a physician or mental-health professional.

References

Allen, R. P. 2004. *Scripts and Strategies in Hypnotherapy: The Complete Works*. Bancyfelin, Wales: Crown House.

Allison, D. B., and M. S. Faith. 1996. Hypnosis as an adjunct to cognitive behavioral psychotherapy for obesity: A meta-analytical appraisal. *Journal of Consulting and Clinical Psychology* 64 (3): 513–16.

Amen, D. G., and L. C. Routh. 2004. *Healing Anxiety and Depression*. New York: Berkeley Books.

American Cancer Society. 2006. Calculate your daily calorie needs. Available online at <www.cancer.org/docroot/PED/content/PED_6_1x_Calorie_Calculator.asp?sitearea=&level=>.

American Society of Bariatric Physicians. 2005. Frequently asked questions. Available online at <www.asbp.org/faq.asp>.

Andersen, M. S. 1985. Hypnotizability as a factor in the hypnotic treatment of obesity. *International Journal of Clinical and Experimental Hypnosis* 33 (2): 150–59.

Andreas, C. 1992. *Advanced Language Patterns*. [Audiotape]. Boulder, CO: NLP Comprehensive.

Andreas, C., and S. Andreas. 1989. *Heart of the Mind*. Moab, UT: Real People Press.

Andreas, C., and T. Andreas. 1991. Aligning perceptual positions: A new distinction in NLP. *Anchor Point*, February, 1–6.

Andreas, C., and T. Andreas. 1994. *Core Transformation: Reaching the Wellspring Within*. Moab, UT: Real People Press.

Bandler, R. 1985. *Using Your Brain for a Change*. Moab, UT: Real People Press.

Bandler, R. 1993. *Time for A Change*. Cupertino, CA: Meta Publications.

Bandler, R., and J. Grinder. 1979. *Frogs Into Princes*. Moab, UT: Real People Press.

Bandler, R., and J. Grinder. 1982. *Reframing: Neuro-Linguistic Programming and the Transformation of Meaning*. Moab, UT: Real People Press.

Bannister, E. W., and S. R. Brown. 1968. The relative energy requirements of physical activity. In H. B. Falls, ed., *Exercise Physiology*. New York: Academic Press.

Barabasz, M., and D. Spiegel. 1989. Hypnotizability and weight loss in obese subjects. *International Journal of Eating Disorders* 8: 335–41.

Battino, R. 2000. *Guided Imagery and Other Approaches to Healing*. Bancyfelin, Wales: Crown House.

Beaulieu, D. 2003. *Eye Movement Integration Therapy*. Bancyfelin, Wales: Crown House.

Bodenhamer, B. G. 2004. *Mastering Blocking and Stuttering*. Bancyfelin, Wales: Crown House.

Bodenhamer, B. G., and L. M. Hall. 1997a. *Figuring Out People: Design Engineering with Meta-programs*. Bancyfelin, Wales: Crown House.

Bodenhamer, B. G., and L. M. Hall. 1997b. *Time Lining: Patterns for Adventuring in Time*. Bancyfelin, Wales: Crown House.

Bolocofsky, D. N., D. Spinier, and L. Coulthard-Morris. 1985. Effectiveness of hypnosis as an adjunct to behavioral weight management. *Journal of Clinical Psychology* 41 (1): 35–41.

Burton, J., and B. G. Bodenhamer. 2000. *Hypnotic Language: Its Structure and Use*. Bancyfelin, Wales: Crown House.

Centers for Disease Control and Prevention. 2006. BMI—body mass index: About BMI for adults. Available online at <www.cdc.gov/ nccdphp/dnpa/bmi/adult_BMI/ about_adult_BMI.htm>.

Charvet, S. R. 1995. *Words That Change Minds: Mastering the Language of Influence*. Dubuque, IA: Kendall/Hunt.

Citrenbaum, C. M., M. E. King, and W. I. Cohen. 1985. *Modern Clinical Hypnosis for Habit Control*. New York: W. W. Norton.

Cochrane, G. 1992. Hypnosis and weight reduction: Which is the cart and which is the horse? *American Journal of Clinical Hypnosis* 35 (2): 109–18.

Cochrane, G., and J. Friesen. 1986. Hypnotherapy in weight loss treatment. *Journal of Consulting and Clinical Psychology* 54: 489–92.

Coman, C., and B. Evans. 1995. Clinical update on eating disorders and obesity: Implications for treatment with hypnosis. *Australian Journal of Clinical and Experimental Hypnosis* 23 (1): 1–13.

Connelly, J. 2004. *Life Change Conversations: The Power of Transformational Conversation*. Jupiter, FL: Institute for Survivors of Sexual Violence.

Connelly, J. 2005. *Dynamic Hypnotherapy and Rapid Trauma Resolution*. Jupiter, FL: Institute for Survivors of Sexual Violence.

Corsetty, K., and J. Pearson. 2000. *Healthy Habits: Total Conditioning for a Healthy Body and Mind*. Lincoln, NE: Dageforde Press.

de Shazer, S. 1988. *Clues: Investigating Solutions in Brief Therapy*. New York: W. W. Norton.

Dilts, R. 1990. *Changing Belief Systems with NLP*. Cupertino, CA: Meta Publications.

Dilts, R., and J. DeLozier. 2000. *The Encyclopedia of Systemic NLP and NLP New Coding*. Scotts Valley, CA: NLP University Press.

Emmerson, G. 2003. *Ego State Therapy*. Bancyfelin, Wales: Crown House.

Expert Group Convened by Health Promotion Directorate. 1988. *Canadian Guidelines for Healthy Weights.* Ottawa: Health and Welfare Canada, Health Services and Promotion Branch.

Farrington, G. 1985. Effects of self-hypnosis audiotapes on weight loss: Relationship with ego-strength, motivation, anxiety, and locus of control. *Dissertation Abstracts International* 46 (6B): 2048.

Fraser, L. 1997. The diet trap. *Family Therapy Networker,* May–June. Available online at <www.FamilyTherapyNetworker.com>.

Gangwisch, J., and S. Heymsfield. 2004. Lack of sleep may lead to excess weight. Paper presented to the North American Association for the Study of Obesity Annual Scientific Meeting, November 14–18, 2004, Las Vegas, NV.

Gordon, D. 1978. *Therapeutic Metaphors.* Cupertino, CA: Meta Publications.

Greaves, E., G. Tidy, and R. A. S. Christie. 1995. Hypnotherapy and weight loss. *Nutrition and Food Science* 95 (6).

Grodski, L. 2000. *Building Your Ideal Private Practice.* New York: W. W. Norton.

Haley, J. 1984. *Ordeal Therapy: Unusual Ways to Change Behavior.* San Francisco, CA: Jossey-Bass.

Hall, L. M. 1995. *The Spirit of NLP.* Bancyfelin, Wales: Crown House.

Hall, L. M. 2000. *Frame Games: Advanced Persuasion Skills.* Clifton, CO: Empowerment Technologies, E. T. Publications.

Hall, L. M. 2001. *Games Slim People Play.* Grand Junction, CO: Neuro-Semantics.

Hall, L. M., and B. Belnap. 2004. *The Sourcebook of Magic: A Comprehensive Guide to NLP Change Patterns.* 2nd ed. Bancyfelin, Wales: Crown House.

Hall, L. M., and B. G. Bodenhamer. 1999a. *The Structure of Excellence.* Grand Junction, CO: Empowerment Technologies/E. T. Publications.

Hall, L. M., and B. G. Bodenhamer. 1999b. *The User's Manual for the Brain.* Vol. 1. Clifton, CO: Neuro-Semantics.

Hall, L. M., and B. G. Bodenhamer. 2001a. *Games for Mastering Fear.* Clifton, CO: Neuro-Semantics.

Hall, L. M., and B. G. Bodenhamer. 2001b. *Mind Lines: Lines for Changing Minds.* 4th ed. Clifton, CO: Neuro-Semantics.

Hall, L. M., and B. G. Bodenhamer. 2003. *The User's Manual for the Brain.* Vol. 2. Bancyfelin, Wales: Crown House.

Harris, C. 1999. *Think Yourself Slim: A Unique Approach to Weight Loss.* Shaftesbury, Dorset, and Boston, MA: Element.

Hunt, M. 1984. Self-hypnosis works! *Reader's Digest,* April, 164–68.

James, T., L. Flores, and J. Schober. 2000. *Hypnosis: A Comprehensive Guide*. Bancyfelin, Wales: Crown House.

James, T., and W. Woodsmall. 1988. *Time Line Therapy and the Basis of Personality*. Cupertino, CA: Meta Publications.

Kane, S., and K. Olness. 2004. *The Art of Therapeutic Communication: The Collected Works of Kay F. Thompson*. Bancyfelin, Wales: Crown House.

Kirsch, I., G. Montgomery, and G. Sapirstein. 1995. Hypnosis as an adjunct to cognitive-behavioral weight loss treatments—Another meta-reanalysis. *Journal of Consulting and Clinical Psychology* 63: 214–20.

Lankton, S. and C. Lankton. 1990. *Metaphor: Elements and Construction*. Paper from a workshop presented at the Third Eastern Conference on Ericksonian Hypnosis and Psychotherapy, Philadelphia, PA, 1992.

Lankton, S., and C. Lankton. 1983. *The Answer Within: A Clinical Framework of Ericksonian Hypnotherapy*. New York: Brunner/Mazel.

McDermott, I., and W. Jago. 2001. *The NLP Coach*. London: Piatkus.

McDonald, R. 1979. *The Walking Belief Change Pattern*. Boulder, CO: NLP Comprehensive.

McGowan, K. 2004. Addiction: Pay attention. *Psychology Today*, Nov.–Dec. Available online: Document ID 3571 <http://www.psychologytoday.com/articles/pto-3571.html>.

Merlevede, P. E., and D. C. Bridoux. 2003. *Mastering Mentoring and Coaching with Emotional Intelligence*. Bancyfelin, Wales: Crown House.

Mignot, E., S. Taheri, L. Lin, and T. Young. 2004. Stanford study links obesity to hormonal changes from lack of sleep. *Public Library of Science*, Dec. 8, 2004. Summarized on Stanford University Medical Center, Office of Communication and Public Affairs web site at <http://news-service.stanford.edu/news/2004/december8/med-sleep-1208.html>.

Morrill, D. H. 2000. *Great Escapes*. Vol. 2: *Assisting Adults and Youth to Obtain What They Desire*. Tacoma, WA: New Beginnings.

Overdurf, J., and J. Silverthorn. 1995. Recovering options: The transformation of addictive processes. *Anchor Point*, June, 29–35.

Passmore, R., and J. V. G. A. Dumin. 1955. Human energy expenditure. *Physiological Reviews* 35: 801.

Preston, M. D. 2001. *Hypnosis: Medicine of the Mind*. Tempe, AZ: Dandelion Books.

Schaumberg L. L. et al. 1995. Hypnosis as a clinical intervention for weight reduction and self-esteem improvement in young women. *International Journal of Psychiatric Nursing Research* 1 (3): 99–107.

Speigel, H. 1972. An eye-roll test for hypnotizability. *American Journal of Clinical Hypnosis* 15: 25–28.

Stern, D., H. Speigel, and J. Nee. 1979. The Hypnotic Induction Profile: Normative observations, reliability, and validity. *American Journal of Clinical Hypnosis* 31: 109–32.

Stradling, J., D. Roberts, and F. Lovelock. 1998. Controlled trial of hypnotherapy for weight loss in patients with obstructive sleep apnea. *International Journal of Obesity* 22: 278–81.

Taheri, S. 2004. The mechanisms for the interaction between sleep and metabolism. Available online at the University of Bristol, Laboratories for Integrative Neuroscience and Endocrinology web site at <www.bris.ac.uk/Depts/URCN/>.

Vanderlinden, J., and W. Vandereycken. 1994. The (limited) possibilities of hypnotherapy in the treatment of obesity. *American Journal of Clinical Hypnosis* 36 (4): 248–57.

Waldholz, M. 2003. Altered states: Hypnosis goes mainstream. *Wall Street Journal*, October 7, Personal Health section.

Weight-control Information Network. 2005. Statistics related to overweight and obesity. Available online at <http://win.niddk.nih.gov/statistics/index.htm>.

Weitzenhoffer, A., and E. Hilgard. 1963. *Stanford Profile Scales of Hypnotic Susceptibility*, Forms I and II. Palo Alto, CA: Consulting Psychologists Press.

Whitworth, L., H. Kimsey-House, and P. Sandahl. 1998. *Co-active Coaching*. Palo Alto, CA: Davies-Black.

World Health Organization. 1998. *Obesity: Preventing and Managing the Global Epidemic*. WHO Technical Report Series. Geneva: WHO.

Yapko, M. 1990. *Trancework: An Introduction to the Practice of Clinical Hypnosis*. New York: Brunner/Mazel.

The Weight, Hypnotherapy and YOU

Weight Reduction Program

Client Workbook

Judith E. Pearson, Ph.D.

Contents

WHY Client Workbook © 2006 Crown House Publishing, www.CHPUS.com, www.crownhouse.co.uk

Introduction

Welcome to the *Weight, Hypnotherapy and YOU (WHY) Weight Reduction Program Client Workbook*. The WHY Program was designed for people just like you who sincerely want to reduce their weight and are willing to make lasting lifestyle changes to reach and maintain their preferred weight.

The eight sessions of the WHY Program were developed by Dr. Judy Pearson, a licensed professional counselor, master trainer, practitioner of Neuro-Linguistic Programming (NLP), and a master clinical hypnotherapist. These eight sessions are to be administered by a certified hypnotherapist and NLP practitioner. Dr. Pearson developed the program based on interviews and therapy sessions with numerous clients who struggled with weight reduction, interviewing people who had successfully reached their goal weight and consulting with nurses, nutritionists, motivational coaches, social workers, counselors, and psychologists. Ideas for the program also came from NLP books mentioned throughout these assignments.

These assignments are intended to complement the work you do with your practitioner. Each assignment focuses on a specific cognitive skill, a mindset if you will, related to successful weight control. Each assignment will contribute to your success, so give each one your full attention and motivation. If you have any questions or concerns about any assignment, be sure to discuss them with your practitioner.

Program Overview

In session 1, "Intake Interview and Introduction to the WHY Program," you'll have an interview with your practitioner and get an overview of the WHY Program. The accompanying assignment, "Get the Results You Want: Well-Formed Outcomes for Weight Control," teaches you how to create well-formed outcomes that are specific and motivating.

In session 2, "Reframing Compulsive Eating," you'll complete a process to examine some of your unconscious motives behind overeating, and the assignment helps you examine the difference between "Trim-Slim Thinking versus Fat Thinking."

In session 3, "Training in Self-Hypnosis," you'll learn self-hypnosis, and the assignment is a series of worksheets, or templates, that help you design your own self-hypnosis sessions in "Learning Self-Hypnosis: The Seven-Step Self-Hypnosis Process."

Session 4, "Stopping Emotional Eating with Stress Management," teaches you stress management tools to curb the eating for comfort that sometimes accompanies stress. The assignment, "Stress Management and Emotional Eating," discusses ways to stress-proof your life, manage stress in healthy ways, and reverse the addiction to emotional eating. The accompanying bonus report, "Boost Your Brain to Curb Compulsive Eating!" gives you brain-health recommendations that may help you improve your eating patterns.

Session 5, "Making Sensible Food Choices," is a hypnotherapy session focusing on choosing healthful, nutritious, slenderizing foods. The hypnotherapy portion is audio recorded for you to use on your own at home. The assignment calls for you to designate healthful and not-so-healthful foods and complete "A Two-Week Food Diary," so that you become more aware of your eating patterns.

Session 6, "Creating an Intelligent Relationship with Food," is another recorded hypnotherapy session encouraging you to eat when you are hungry and stop eating when you are full. The assignment teaches you a step-by-step process called "The NLP Slender Eating Strategy."

Session 7, "Boosting Motivation to Exercise," is a recorded hypnotherapy session that revs up your motivation to exercise. The accompanying bonus report, "The Benefits of Exercise," tells you how exercise can help you and how to get started on a safe, healthy exercise program. The "Mind Management" assignment will help you prepare for session 8.

Session 8, "Pulling It All Together for Lasting Results," is a recorded hypnotherapy session that encourages you to take your mindset into the future so that the changes you've made are lasting. The assignment is called "Keep Going: Make Changes Last, Make Motivation Last."

After session 8, you may want to return for additional follow-up sessions with your practitioner, to work through any other issues that may be interfering with the success you seek. You might want to talk about relationships, limiting beliefs, self-esteem, work-related problems, time management, relationships, or perhaps family-related concerns—anything that will help you reduce stress, love yourself, and maintain your progress.

Part of your agreement to participate in the WHY Program is that you select a nutrition plan approved or recommended by a physician, nurse, or nutritionist. While you are in the WHY Program, be sure to stick with your nutrition plan diligently, weigh yourself regularly to keep track of your progress, follow any guidelines established by your physician, get adequate rest, and choose an exercise plan to implement by session 7. If you encounter any problems or difficulties, discuss them with your practitioner so that he or she can modify the program, where appropriate, to meet your needs.

The task you have undertaken is not easy. It is time-consuming and life-changing, and you are worth it. You have what it takes. Believe in yourself and see the results!

Assignment for Session 1

Get the Results You Want: Well-Formed Outcomes for Weight Control

What if you could have a healthy body, feeling attractive, fit, and full of vitality? How would you look? How would you feel? What rewards and satisfactions would you enjoy? What habits would you pursue on a daily basis? What would you be doing now that you haven't done in the past? How could your life be different? You *know* the answers to these questions. Go ahead and create your dream! Close your eyes and live it. Be there now. Dream the dream, and let the dream become like a magnet that pulls you into the future. Make it just the way you want it. Imagine it in detail. Make it compellingly real. Take it all in and enjoy it. Believe in your possibilities!

- Is it worth making some changes in your priorities?
- Is it worth the effort to learn some new ways of selecting foods?
- Is it worth taking the time to exercise on a regular basis?
- Is it worth giving up some limiting beliefs and bad habits and excuses?
- Is it worth learning how to love and take care of yourself?

Put Your Vision into Words

Now that you've visualized your future, the next step is to put it into words. Words and pictures are the building materials of our thoughts, emotions, and behaviors. Words are the basis of our self-talk—the way we mentally speak to ourselves. The quality of your self-talk can influence your success. Positive, enthusiastic self-talk evokes positive emotions and motivation. Negative, self-critical, or pessimistic self-talk leads to depression and lassitude.

By putting what you want into words, you are formulating an outcome—a statement of what you intend to accomplish. Words are the primary tools we use to program our emotions and behaviors, so it's important to select powerful, effective words when formulating an outcome. Why? A poorly formed outcome steers your brain in the wrong direction and keeps you stuck. A well-formed outcome, on the other hand, boosts your motivation and gets your brain working toward real results and solutions. A well-formed outcome is

A-1

especially important when your outcome requires ongoing commitment and extensive lifestyle changes—like when you decide to modify eating habits and start exercising in order to achieve and maintain a healthy weight.

In the popular best-seller *The Seven Habits of Highly Effective People* (Simon and Schuster, 1989), author Stephen Covey advised readers to "begin with the end in mind." Any endeavor starts with a clearly stated objective. You won't get anywhere unless you know where you are going. A well-formed outcome is the first step toward success. The concept comes from Neuro-Linguistic Programming (NLP), and counselors, coaches, psychologists, and social workers use it to help their clients establish and reach workable goals and realize their dreams and ambitions. If you want to make a change for the better, start with a well-formed outcome. The well-formed outcome begins with a simple question: "What do you want?"

Here are seven guidelines for creating empowering outcomes that will strengthen your commitment to making the changes that will lead to a lifetime of fitness and health.

1. State Your Outcome in the Positive

Start with what you want, not what you don't want. Instead of, "I want to stop eating junk food," say, "I eat fruits and vegetables every day." If you create outcomes around what you do *not* want, you continue to focus on the problem, rather than directing your thoughts toward the solution. If you are thinking of what you *don't* want, your unconscious mind is creating an image of the very thing you want to avoid, and you will be unconsciously drawn toward it. For example, if someone says to you, "Do *not* think about a purple tree," what is the first thing that comes to your mind? —A purple tree, of course! Start programming your mind for what you want, because you can never get enough of what you *don't* want.

Moreover, once you've formulated the outcome you choose, stop thinking about it as something you *want*. Instead, start thinking about it as something you have now or are creating now. The subconscious mind can be very literal. When you say "I want …" your subconscious mind hears "I lack …" To want something is to lack that thing. To create your outcome, speak of it as though you have it now, you choose to have it now, and you are creating it now.

2. State Your Outcome in the Present Tense

Your outcomes are about what you are doing now and into future, regardless of what has happened in the past. Although it makes perfect sense that outcomes are about now and the future, some people continue to dwell on the past when thinking about what they want. Statements like, "I wish I had been a thin teenager" or "I should have learned how to eat properly by now" are not well-formed outcomes. You can't change the past, so put your attention and energies on what you can accomplish today, tomorrow, and from now on.

State your outcomes in the present tense, not the future tense. If you say "I will eat nutritious foods," your subconscious mind hears "I will" and assumes the new behavior will occur sometime later, in the future, rather than now. By putting your outcome in the present tense, you notify your subconscious mind that your outcomes and new behaviors are taking place NOW!

3. Create Your Goals around Your Own Behaviors and Feelings

Only you can create your future. No one else can do it for you. Make certain that your outcomes are about changing your own emotions and behaviors, not about what someone else wants you to do, or what you want someone else to do. Statements like, "My spouse goes to the gym with me" or "My friends compliment me on my new figure" won't work. Granted, your outcomes *could* include the steps you are taking to influence the behavior of those around you, and you *could* improve your communication skills to get more cooperation from others. Just remember, you cannot control others, so don't base your success on what they do. Make your outcomes self-initiated and about you.

4. State Your Outcomes in Specific Terms

Our minds code outcomes as accomplishable when those outcomes are stated (and visualized) specifically. Specific outcomes are about observable, measurable behaviors and clearly defined emotional states. Make your outcomes specific by stating when, where, and how often you want them. Avoid vague words like "more," "less," or "some." Instead of "I am doing better," say "I plan my meals, eat nutritious foods, and at least every other day, I ride a stationary bike." Can you feel the difference between those two statements? The second one feels more doable, exact, and real, doesn't it?

5. Make Your Outcomes Realistic and Achievable

Be careful about overblown or exaggerated outcomes. If they inspire you, that's fine. But if they lead to disappointment, procrastination, and frustration, then set your sights on something more realistic and achievable. We'd all like to make a million dollars a year, be in good enough shape to run a marathon, and look like some fashion model or movie star, but for many of us, it's difficult to

WHY Client Workbook © 2006 Crown House Publishing, www.CHPUS.com, www.crownhouse.co.uk

really see ourselves doing those things—or to really know whether those things are possible.

Maybe it's better to channel your energies into simply reaching a healthy weight and sticking with intelligent meal planning. Make your time frames realistic. Give your body sufficient time to make adjustments. With weight reduction, shedding only one or two pounds a week is healthy. If you are just starting an exercise program, start out with short, easy workouts and gradually build your strength and stamina to avoid overfatigue, injury, or inflammation to muscles and joints.

6. State Your Outcomes without Equivocation

Equivocation is a hedge—it says "I'm willing to fail" or "I don't really want to." Avoid halfhearted statements like "Well, I guess I might exercise some more when I get around to it." Halfhearted statements are not motivating; they make you yawn! A well-formed outcome is stated affirmatively, without any hemming and hawing.

7. Make Your Outcomes Congruent with Who You Are

An *"ecological"* outcome is safe and realistic for your situation, and doesn't conflict with your needs or values. If you choose an outcome that isn't ecological, it won't feel right. You won't stick with it, or you'll engage in self-sabotage. Don't commit to any outcome until you've checked in with yourself—consulted your inner wisdom, so to speak—about whether you can truly commit to this course of action. If you feel vaguely uncomfortable about some outcome you've decided on, then there is probably some issue you need to resolve—or you may need to modify the outcome. Ask yourself, "Am I willing to do what it takes?" and "Is it worth it?" Every significant life choice carries a cost, a sacrifice, or a trade-off. Each new commitment you make means you will forfeit other choices and opportunities.

Choose Your Chunk Size

"Chunk size" is an important motivation factor in how you define an outcome. Chunk size is your perception of whether your outcome seems too large to undertake, too small to be significant, or just right so that it seems doable and worthwhile.

If your outcome is well-formed but seems daunting or overwhelming, you are thinking too big. Chunk your outcome down to doable steps. Instead of "I'm

WHY Client Workbook © 2006 Crown House Publishing, www.CHPUS.com, www.crownhouse.co.uk

losing forty pounds by Christmas," say, "I'm losing two pounds a week by following this daily meal plan."

If your outcome is well-formed but seems insignificant or not worthwhile, you are thinking too small. Chunk up to see the bigger picture and long-term, cumulative benefits and meanings that tie in with your values. Instead of, "So what if I lose two pounds this week? What does it matter? I'll still be fat," say, "If I lose two pounds this week, I can do the same next week and each week, and in three months I'll be twenty-four pounds slimmer, and I'll fit into a size 10 in time for the class reunion! I'll feel so attractive and confident, I'll glow!" Got it? Keep your eye on the prize!

Sacrifices or Trade-offs?

Any worthwhile goal entails some difficulty, sustained effort, and trade-offs. You might call these sacrifices, but the trade-off is really giving up a short-term satisfaction in favor of something else that is more valuable, enduring, and ultimately more fulfilling. Some people call this delayed gratification, but I have a more elegant word for it: *discipline.*

Learning to say *no* to old habits can be difficult until the old habit is extinguished and a new one takes its place. You could, for example, spend less time on the computer in order to find time to exercise. You could snack on fresh vegetables instead of potato chips. To make a trade-off requires two skills: (1) minimizing the importance of whatever you are giving up or cutting back on, and (2) keeping the larger picture (your vision) in mind. Be careful in the way you talk to yourself. You can say, "Oh no! I have to give up ice cream and suffer for the rest of my life!" But that statement will only undermine your commitment, because it exaggerates the displeasure of having no ice cream. This tactic is called *catastrophizing.* Instead say, "What's a little ice cream compared to the freedom and confidence of a healthy, slim figure?" As you say these words, call your vision to mind—a glowing, Technicolor image of a healthy, active you. Remind yourself that the results are well worth the trade-offs.

Activity: Put It in Writing

Now that you've defined your outcomes, write them out. A study of the 1953 graduates of Yale University clearly demonstrates the importance of committing goals to paper. The graduates were interviewed and asked if they had a clear, specific set of goals written down, along with a plan for achieving those goals. Only 3 percent had such written goals. Twenty years later, in 1973, the researchers went back and interviewed the surviving members of the 1953

WHY Client Workbook © 2006 Crown House Publishing, www.CHPUS.com, www.crownhouse.co.uk

graduating class. They discovered that the 3 percent with specific, written goals were worth more in financial terms than the other 97 percent combined!

Below, write outcomes that describe the changes you want to make in order to develop a healthy lifestyle, so that you reach and maintain your target weight:

1. _____

2. _____

3. _____

4. _____

Now close your eyes, step into each of these outcomes, and live it in your mind. Imagine doing it. Anticipate your thoughts and feelings. Imagine the satisfaction you feel as you fulfill each one. See the short-term and long-term rewards. Put these outcomes on index cards and carry them with you during the day, so that you can read them and remind yourself where you are going. Tape your outcomes to your refrigerator or the mirror on your dresser, so that you see them often and keep them in the forefront of your mind. Put them in your PDA or keep them handy on your computer desktop.

This week, take a piece of clothing from your closet, something that is a size you used to wear—and, if possible, is your ideal size: a pair of slacks or skirt or dress or maybe even a swimsuit. Make sure this item of clothing is attractive and something you'd like to wear again. Place this item on a hanger and put it on your closet door, bedroom door, bathroom door, or someplace where you are likely to see it often. Every time you see it, visualize yourself wearing it and feeling proud. Let it remind you that you have what it takes to achieve your perfect size.

Next Steps

Now that you have well-formed outcomes, you can advance into the planning stages by asking additional questions:

- How am I going to do it? What are the steps and the timetable for completion?
- What questions do I have? Do I need more information? Where will I find it?
- What are my action steps? How often will I engage in these actions?
- Who else will be involved, and what do I want them to do?
- How will I know I am making progress?
- Once I have the result I want, how do I maintain it, make it even better, or decide when it's time to go on to another outcome?

Go for It!

Now that you know how to create well-formed outcomes, go for it! Don't let negative, depressing, or pessimistic thoughts talk you out of it. Decide that you are going to have your chosen outcome, don't take no for an answer, and commit to the outcome with passion, drive, and motivation. Think positively and optimistically. Be ready to meet challenges with courage and creativity, setbacks with persistence, and problems with solutions. Ask for help when you need it. Be unstoppable! State your well-formed outcomes and bring them into reality!

Portions of this assignment were excerpted and adapted from Healthy Habits: Total Conditioning for a Healthy Body and Mind, *by Kathy Corsetty and Judith E. Pearson (Lincoln, NE: Dageforde Press, 2000).*

Assignment for Session 2

Trim-Slim Thinking versus Fat Thinking

Do you practice Fat Thinking, or do you practice Trim-Slim Thinking? When compared to people who have weight problems, people who find it easy to stay trim and slim seem to have a different way of thinking about food and weight management. By becoming aware of those differences, you may decide to adapt some new thinking patterns.[1]

Overweight people tend to find comfort in food. Trim-Slim people, by contrast, seldom look to food for comfort when experiencing difficult emotions. In fact, sometimes stress actually diminishes their appetite! They might say, "I'm too upset to eat!" They have other strategies for coping with stress, such as confiding in a friend, gathering information, and mapping out a plan of action. When they get stuck in unwanted emotions, they seldom soothe themselves with food. They choose other soothing activities, such as listening to music, taking a hot bath, going for a walk, or journaling.

Fat Thinking says, "I'll eat now, because I may be hungry later." People who are naturally slender eat when they feel hungry. They eat for one meal at a time, without thinking ahead to the next meal. Sure they might feel hungry later, but they don't mind feeling a little hungry now and then. If they need to keep up their energy and blood sugar levels throughout the day, they carry healthful snacks with them wherever they go, so that they won't be tempted to eat junk foods.

Overweight people may eat due to external cues—such as seeing an advertisement about food, seeing other people eat, smelling food, or seeing food. The Trim-Slim person eats in response to bodily cues indicating hunger. Those cues might be a hollow feeling in the stomach; a tired feeling or difficulty concentrating, which indicates a need for an energy boost; or a taste sensation in the mouth, indicating a desire for a specific flavor of food—salty, savory, sweet, or sour. Sometimes they drink a glass of water before deciding whether they are truly hungry, to avoid confusing hunger with thirst.

---

1. Excess weight is not caused solely by psychological factors. Other factors—such as body chemistry, genetics, allergies, metabolic and endocrine deficiencies, and a host of other physical ailments—can contribute. Seek your physician's advice and have a complete physical examination before undertaking any weight management program.

A-9

Fat Thinking leads to eating beyond the point of satiety. Some overweight people say they eat too fast, they don't think about how much they are eating, and they are not aware of what feeling full is like. One way to be Trim and Slim is to eat slowly and with consciousness, being aware that the average adult human stomach can hold only about two heaping handfuls of food (about the size of a small cantaloupe) and being very much aware of that stuffy, heavy fullness in the stomach that indicates the point of satiety. At that point, a Trim-Slim eater does not want another bite, no matter how good the food tastes, because an overstuffed stomach feels like having a boulder in the belly.

Do you ever binge on foods that are loaded with calories, sugar, or fat because "I just can't stop at one or two?" Afterwards do you feel regret? A Trim-Slim eater can stop at "just a bite or two" and consider that a satisfying indulgence.

Fat Thinking endows food with meaning. For example, "Cheeseburgers are my downfall" or "Mashed potatoes and gravy are my comfort food" or "Chocolate is my friend" or "The cookies in the cupboard are calling to me." To a Trim-Slim person, saying such things is utter nonsense. It would never occur to a Trim and Slim person to say such things about food, because food "is just something you eat when you feel hungry—otherwise, it's no big deal."

Some overweight folks avoid getting on the bathroom scale because they get depressed when they see how much they weigh, and they feel bad about themselves. This is often how their weight got out of control in the first place—because they didn't keep track of those extra pounds. Trim-Slim people weigh themselves at regular intervals, to check on any extra pounds that might be sneaking up on them. They also monitor how their clothes fit to stay aware of weight changes. They take action at the first indication of those few extra pounds by cutting back on some high-calorie foods, skipping a few snacks, substituting low-calorie foods and drinks, and getting more exercise than usual. To a Trim-Slim person, the bathroom scale is a dependable source of feedback and a vital tool for weight management. Numbers don't lie! A Trim-Slim person would tell you that not checking the bathroom scale is like driving a car without a gas gauge or a speedometer!

Probably the number-one cognitive factor that contributes to being overweight is denial. When the weight starts creeping up, overweight people tend to go into denial until the excess weight is a significant problem that can no longer be ignored. Denial takes the form of statements such as:

- I thought it was normal to put on weight after pregnancy.
- When I saw the extra pounds on the scale, I just assumed my scale was broken, so I threw it out.
- When my jeans got too tight, I thought they had shrunk in the washing machine.

- I kept telling myself a few extra pounds wouldn't matter, and no one would notice.
- I consoled myself with the fact that I wasn't as fat as other people I knew.
- I kept telling myself that putting on weight is a natural side-effect of getting older.

Trim-Slim people know exactly what they want to weigh, and when the scale shows they have exceeded that number—even by only two or three pounds—they take action immediately.

Begin now to think, eat, and live your life as a Trim-Slim person, by adopting some of the preceding thought and behavior patterns. Try one on this week and find out if it works for you. Maybe you are already doing a few of these things, and seeing the results as those extra pounds begin to disappear and you get in touch with the Trim-Slim side of yourself. Doing so isn't easy—it requires revisions in the things you think about, the things you become aware of, and the things you say to yourself. The experts who write advice columns will tell you it takes anywhere from twenty-one to forty days of repetition to install a new habit. Get started now!

Assignment for Session 3

Learning Self-Hypnosis:
The Seven-Step Self-Hypnosis Process

This assignment shows you a seven-step process for designing your own self-hypnosis sessions. Self-hypnosis takes only a few minutes. Find a quiet place where you won't be interrupted. The steps are as follows:

1. Find the blank template in your materials. You can copy the template form to create as many self-hypnosis processes as you wish. Identify the problem you want to address (step 1) and plan it on your template (steps 3–6). (Look at the sample completed templates for examples.)

2. Induce trance. There are many ways to get into a state of focused concentration. Use one that works for you and that you have practiced with your practitioner.

3. Now focus on what you will do as your solution—imagine how you will think, feel, and act.

4. Visualize yourself carrying out the new behavior. This is your mental rehearsal.

5. State positive affirmations that you can easily repeat to yourself to remind yourself about the change you are creating.

6. Now make your own posthypnotic suggestion with this easy formula: "From now on when I encounter X, I do Y."

7. Reorient yourself: open your eyes if they were closed, stretch, and take a deep breath. Done!

Now examine the template examples on the following pages to learn how to create your own self-hypnosis solutions! Then read the rest of the materials to learn how to create your own self-hypnosis audio recordings.

Notice a few things about these examples. They involve the elements of a well-formed *commitment to change*. That is, they contain the following elements:

WHY Client Workbook © 2006 Crown House Publishing, www.CHPUS.com, www.crownhouse.co.uk

1. They focus on the positive—on what you want, not on what you don't want.

2. They remind you to use your inner resources and strengths.

3. They tap into your four sources of *personal power:* what you think, what you feel, what you say, and what you do.

4. The emphasis is on creating a solution, not analyzing the problem.

5. They are future-oriented—no lamenting about the past here.

6. The change is self-initiated—no one else has to do it for you, and you don't have to wait for external circumstances to change first.

7. The solution happens at a certain time and place or under specific circumstances. When you think of the solution, you specify where and when you intend to bring it about. This lends clarity to your thinking, preferable to a vague statement such as "I want to be happier."

8. The templates involve thinking in both words and pictures. What you say to yourself and what you visualize can have powerful impacts on your future actions and feelings.

9. Make or ask your practitioner for as many copies of the blank template as you wish, so that you can design your own self-hypnosis solutions. For each one, complete the worksheet. Then carry out the seven steps, beginning with a definition of the problem, then taking yourself into trance, creating the solution, and ending with reorienting yourself. You can use the methods you have learned for accessing a light trance state whenever it is safe and convenient for you to close your eyes and concentrate for a few minutes. After a while and with practice, the seven steps will flow easily and logically for you, and you will apply them easily and spontaneously.

Another way to hypnotize yourself is with an audio recording of your own voice. You tell yourself to relax, focus your thoughts, close your eyes, and guide yourself through the steps in each template. If you wish to create a self-hypnosis tape for yourself, a sample hypnosis script outline is included in these materials. Just tailor it to your own needs.

Self-hypnosis is a way to program your mind and body for great results! Get a pen or pencil and start designing your own self-hypnosis sessions now! Simply fill in new templates, one by one, as you address each new problem on your way to obtaining your *preferred weight.* Have fun, stay positive, and good luck with your progress!

Sample Self-Hypnosis Template 1

Step 1: Problem or concern: <u>I eat whenever I feel stressed out. Example: when</u>

<u>someone criticizes me.</u>

Step 2: Self-Hypnosis Induction: Take a deep breath and focus your concentration.

Step 3: Create the solution: how you want to respond differently—how you will think, act, and feel.

New thinking: <u>Criticism is only another person's opinion. It is not</u>

<u>necessarily accurate. I can treat it just as information that may or may not</u>

<u>be useful to me.</u>

New feeling: <u>I detach from the criticism so that I can remain objective</u>

<u>about it.</u>

New actions: <u>I respond calmly and tactfully.</u>

Step 4: Visualize yourself carrying out the solution in a situation that previously would have been challenging. This is your mental rehearsal.

<u>I visualize a coworker criticizing one of my reports, saying things I feel</u>

<u>are unfair. I take a deep breath and feel relaxed. I tell myself that the criticism</u>

<u>is only information for me to evaluate. I feel calm and detached. I calmly look at</u>

<u>the coworker and say, "I'll gladly listen to any specific recommendations for</u>

<u>improvement."</u>

Step 5: Your positive affirmations: <u>The calmer I feel, the more I make wise</u>

<u>choices about food.</u>

<u>I am in charge of my own self-esteem, and no one else can take it away from me.</u>

<u>I eat only when I feel hungry.</u>

<u>When I feel stressed out, I seek solutions, not more food!</u>

Step 6: Your posthypnotic suggestion:

From now on whenever I encounter <u>*someone criticizing me*</u>

I <u>*calmly take a deep breath and recall that I am in charge of my self-esteem*</u>

<u>*and feelings. I think clearly and remind myself that I am okay and criticism*</u>

<u>*is only information. I respond calmly and tactfully. I feel good about it*</u>

<u>*afterwards.*</u>

Step 7: Reorient yourself: Open your eyes, stretch, and take a deep breath. Done!

Sample Self-Hypnosis Template 2

Step 1: Problem or concern: *I need to exercise more often.*

Step 2: Self-Hypnosis Induction: Take a deep breath and focus your concentration.

Step 3: Create the solution: how you want to respond differently—how you will think, act, and feel.

New thinking: *I know exercise makes me feel great physically, emotionally, and mentally.*

New feeling: *I feel motivated to exercise. I anticipate it, look forward to it, enjoy it, persist in it, and feel fantastic afterwards.*

New actions: *I schedule a regular time for exercise, and I do it!*

Step 4: Visualize yourself carrying out the solution in a situation that previously would have been challenging. This is your mental rehearsal.

I am in my workout clothes. I am smiling and moving and using my muscles and breathing heavily. I am sweating happily and giving my body a good workout.

I pace myself. I make exercise fun by listening to music or doing it with a friend.

I stick with my routine and honor my exercise time. I feel fantastic afterwards.

I see the results as my conditioning, energy, and stamina improve.

Step 5: Your positive affirmations: *Exercise makes me strong and healthy.*

Exercise helps me lose weight, tone my body, manage stress, build endurance, and increase my personal power.

I enjoy movement and stretching.

I am a physical being, and my body was made to move. I stay fit and firm!

I experience the grace and beauty of a healthy body and a healthy mind.

When it comes to my workout, there are NO EXCUSES!

Step 6: Your posthypnotic suggestion:

From now on whenever I encounter <u>*my scheduled exercise time*</u>

I <u>*suit up, feeling powerful and excited. I take deep breaths and stretch. As*</u>

<u>*I begin my workout, I move at my own pace. As I continue, I feel happy about*</u>

<u>*my increasing strength and flexibility. Even sweat and heavy breathing tell*</u>

<u>*me I am doing something good for myself! I feel pride that I am taking care*</u>

<u>*of my body in this way. I continue to move through my routine, giving myself*</u>

<u>*encouragement to go on. As I cool down, I feel satisfaction with my effort.*</u>

<u>*Afterwards, I feel great, and my entire day seems to go better.*</u>

Step 7: Reorient yourself: Open your eyes, stretch, and take a deep breath. Done!

Sample Self-Hypnosis Template 3

Step 1: Problem or concern: *I eat the wrong kinds of foods. I like sweets and and sugary foods.*

Step 2: Self-Hypnosis Induction: Take a deep breath and focus your concentration.

Step 3: Create the solution: how you want to respond differently—how you will think, act, and feel.

New thinking: *I realize that sweets are loaded with useless calories that drain my energy. I am aware that veggies and fruits are more to my liking and more healthful.*

New feeling: *I feel disinterest in sweets. I feel attracted to fruit and vegetables.*

New actions: *I see sweets and say, "No way! Not in MY body!" I walk right by, ignoring them. I turn them down and choose slenderizing foods instead.*

Step 4: Visualize yourself carrying out the solution in a situation that previously would have been challenging. This is your mental rehearsal.

I am at a party where the buffet table is loaded with sugary foods. I see them and I think, "YUCK! That's fat goo." I choose other foods—healthy foods like fruit—and ignore the bad stuff. I walk right past the desserts, and when I do I feel strong! I feel healthy! I am in control!

Step 5: Your positive affirmations: *I choose healthy foods.*
Sugary, syrupy foods no longer appeal to me. I am attracted to fruits and vegetables instead.
My health and having a toned body are more important than stuffing myself with useless calories.
Nothing is as sweet as a trim body.

Step 6: Your posthypnotic suggestion:

From now on whenever I encounter <u>Sweets—at a party, in the store, at a</u>

<u>picnic, or on a menu or dessert tray</u>

I <u>immediately say YUCK and feel the urge to shun them. I take a deep breath</u>

<u>and ignore them, choosing instead something healthier—such as fruits,</u>

<u>vegetables, or even water. When I do this, I feel a glow of satisfaction,</u>

<u>knowing that I am in control of my food choices.</u>

Step 7: Reorient yourself: Open your eyes, stretch, and take a deep breath. Done!

Sample Self-Hypnosis Template 4

Step 1: Problem or concern: *I despair that I might never reach my preferred weight.*

Step 2: Self-Hypnosis Induction: Take a deep breath and focus your concentration.

Step 3: Create the solution: how you want to respond differently—how you will think, act, and feel.

New thinking: *I decide what, when, and how much I eat. Food is ONLY food, and it has no magical control over me. The formula is simple: eat right and exercise regularly. I can do it! My persistence will pay off! I am entitled to a healthy weight and a fit body, and I am going to have them.*

New feeling: *I feel motivated and empowered.*

New actions: *I continue planning meals and scheduling my exercise times with enthusiasm and determination.*

Step 4: Visualize yourself carrying out the solution in a situation that previously would have been challenging. This is your mental rehearsal.

I maintain a consistent image in my mind of having a healthy, fit, slim body, looking good at my preferred weight. I see myself eating right and exercising regularly day after day. Over time, I feel motivated and excited by this image. I say to myself over and over, "I can do it!"

Step 5: Your positive affirmations: *Eating right and exercising regularly—yes! I can do it!*

My persistence and motivation are leading me to my preferred weight.

Many people have done harder things than this. I will hang in there, and I will triumph!

I have what it takes to achieve my preferred weight!

Step 6: Your posthypnotic suggestion:

From now on whenever I encounter *despairing thoughts about my weight*

I *immediately say to myself, "STOP THAT!" and shake them off. I take a deep*

breath and know that I now feel resolved to have a healthy, trim body. I see

my image of myself at my IDEAL WEIGHT. I repeat my affirmations. I feel

better. I stay motivated and determined to eat right and exercise regularly.

Step 7: Reorient yourself: Open your eyes, stretch, and take a deep breath. Done!

WHY Client Workbook © 2006 Crown House Publishing, www.CHPUS.com, www.crownhouse.co.uk

Self-Hypnosis Template

Step 1: Problem or concern: _____

Step 2: Self-Hypnosis Induction: Take a deep breath and focus your concentration.

Step 3: Create the solution: how you want to respond differently—how you will think, act, and feel.

New thinking: _____

_____

New feeling: _____

_____

New actions: _____

_____

Step 4: Visualize yourself carrying out the solution in a situation that previously would have been challenging. This is your mental rehearsal.

_____

_____

_____

_____

_____

Step 5: Your positive affirmations: _____

_____

_____

_____

_____

_____

A-23

Step 6: Your posthypnotic suggestion:

From now on whenever I encounter _____

I _____

_____

_____

_____

_____

_____

Step 7: Reorient yourself: Open your eyes, stretch, and take a deep breath. Done!

Creating Your Own Self-Hypnosis Audio Recordings

Tailor the following script to your own needs to make your own customized hypnosis audio recordings using the templates in this workbook. Just speak slowly and clearly into the microphone of your tape recorder or audio digital recording device. Helpful instructions are inserted into the script in brackets and italics to guide you. Use the blank templates to describe the changes you want to make and insert steps 3 to 6 from each template into your audio script.

When you prepare to listen to your self-hypnosis recording, find someplace that is quiet and free of distractions. Sit or recline in a comfortable position.

A Sample Script for Self-Hypnosis

Now I take a deep breath and close my eyes. I take another long, deep breath and release all the cares and worries of the day. I take a third deep breath and release all the tension in my muscles, allowing my entire body to relax.

Now I imagine a white board in my mind. I visualize the numbers one to three on the white board. I see the number 1 on the white board. I erase that number 1, and I relax more deeply. I see the number 2 on the white board. I erase that number 2, and I relax even more. I see the number 3 on the white board. I erase that number 3, and I relax more completely than before.

I am using this self-hypnosis session to access my inner strength and wisdom. I am using this self-hypnosis session to solve a problem and create change in my life. The problem I wish to address is:

[*Insert the problem you have identified in step 1 on your template.*]

Now I speak of that problem in the past tense. I let go of that problem. I dismiss it. I put it away from me. It existed only in the past. I am stronger than that problem, and it no longer has any control over me. I now have the solution to that problem, and I am implementing that solution in my daily life so that I think, feel, and act differently.

My new thinking is …

My new feelings are …

My new actions are …

[*For new thinking, feelings, and actions, above, insert the descriptions in step 3 on your template.*]

Now I visualize the changes I am making in my life as I demonstrate new behaviors, thoughts, and feelings in specific contexts and circumstances.

[Describe the short scenario you wrote for step 4 on your template.]

Here is my affirmation that reminds me to stay on track with these beneficial changes ...

[Insert the positive affirmation(s) you chose for step 5 on your template.]

From now on whenever I encounter ... I ...

[Describe the contexts and situations where these new behaviors and to occur, and what you are doing in those circumstances, using what you wrote on your template for step 6.]

I affirm and declare that this change has taken place in my mind and body, and I am improving every day. I am enjoying the rewards and benefits of these new behaviors. I ask my subconscious mind to continue creating this change in a powerful way, making sure this change is lasting and permanent for as long as it serves me and for as long as I desire.

Now I count from 3 to 1, and with each number I become increasingly alert, so that on the number 1, I open my eyes, feeling fully refreshed and alert.

3—coming up now

2—feeling more alert

1—fully alert now, eyes open, ready to continue the day.

[Alternative ending: If you want to listen to your tape before falling asleep at night, omit the previous paragraph and substitute the following one.]

Now I continue to relax, preparing for a deep, peaceful sleep ... a restorative, rejuvenating sleep ... so that I wake up feeling wonderfully refreshed and energized in the morning.

WHY Client Workbook © 2006 Crown House Publishing, www.CHPUS.com, www.crownhouse.co.uk

Assignment for Session 4

Stress Management and Emotional Eating

One factor in excess weight is an association between food and coping with difficult emotions. The emotions that are most difficult to handle are those that arise in response to stressful events and situations. Stress can be a part of normal everyday life: tight deadlines, traffic snarls, mounting paperwork, unruly children, a demanding boss, marital challenges, financial worries—they all lead to stress. Stress is not traumatizing, as is the case with crisis. Nevertheless, stress can wreak havoc on the body and emotions.

Stress is the body's built-in response to any perceived threat. The physical response is an increased heart rate, labored breathing, throbbing temples, muscular tension, and acid in the stomach. With time and repeated exposure, these responses can cause a host of ills such as lowered immunity to infection, ulcers, headaches, hormonal imbalances, and cardiovascular problems.

Stress also brings with it a host of emotions, such as anxiety, anger, fear, depression, inadequacy, confusion, and feelings of being overwhelmed or pressured. Turning to food to alleviate such emotions is known as "emotional eating." Emotional eating is not a response to hunger. It is a response to difficult emotions. Emotional eating is a prominent factor in obesity.

If you have been engaging in emotional eating, there are three things you can do to stop turning to food and to start managing stress in a healthy, mature, sensible manner: (1) stress-proof your life, (2) develop effective stress management skills, and (3) reverse your addiction to food. This assignment will tell you how.

Stress-Proof Your Life

Life is less stressful when you arrange it in such a way that you prevent stress from occurring. No one can live a completely well-ordered, predictable, stress-free life. Nevertheless, there are some things you can do to make life easier:

- Engage in loving, mutually supportive relationships.
- Find meaningful work in an environment you truly enjoy.
- Take care of your health.

A-27

- Learn and apply time-management skills.
- Get organized: bring order to your storage areas, work areas, and paperwork.
- Resolve unfinished business, be done with it, and move on.
- Develop a solution-oriented approach to life's challenges.
- Be willing to learn new things and ask for help when you need it—even if you have to pay for it.

Neglect these responsibilities and guess what happens—more stress!

Develop Effective Stress Management Skills

Stress management skills fall into two general categories: *instrumental* and *palliative*. We apply instrumental skills to change a situation. Using the examples in the first paragraph, healthy ways to change these situations might be, for tight deadlines, to renegotiate the delivery schedule; for traffic jams, to take a new route to the office; for mounting paperwork, to get caught up on it; for child-rearing challenges, to take a parenting class; for a challenging boss, to transfer to another department or get a different job; for marital challenges, to get marriage counseling; and for financial worries to consult a financial planner. Unhealthy ways to change the situation might include coercing others, refusing or avoiding responsibility, or resorting to illegal actions—all of which may eventually make the situation worse, not better.

When we can do nothing to change a situation—or when we aren't willing to change the situation—then we turn to palliative coping skills to alleviate, albeit temporarily perhaps, the uncomfortable emotions associated with it. Healthful ways to soothe difficult emotions might include taking time off, getting a massage, talking things over with a trusted confidant, taking a walk, meditating, praying, listening to music, reading poetry, journaling, taking a hot shower, or getting a good night's sleep. These activities allow the body to restore normal functioning for a while. For people with insufficient coping skills, self-medicating is the palliative alternative. Self-medicating is an unhealthy way of temporarily changing one's emotional state. Favorite candidates are food, sex, alcohol, caffeine, nicotine, or other drugs. These choices reliably change body chemistry, often bringing about pleasurable sensations—all of which may eventually make the situation worse, and all of which hold the potential for addiction.

Now is when you might say, "Addiction? Wait a minute! Are you saying food is addictive?" Yes, when it is used to alleviate emotions. In his book *First Things First* (Simon and Schuster, 1994), Stephen Covey defined addiction as any experience that

- creates predictable, reliable sensations

- becomes the person's primary focus and absorbs attention, taking up increasing amounts of time
- provides an artificial sense of power, control, security, intimacy, or accomplishment
- exacerbates the problems and feelings the person is seeking to remedy
- decreases the person's ability to function properly and damages relationships
- always involves elements of denial and is supported by defense mechanisms

Add to the list: Addictions are progressive in nature and lead to pathology (dysfunctional behavior or emotional instability or health problems or all of these). Do some things on this list begin to sound familiar? The rate of obesity in Western nations shows that food is increasingly the "drug of choice" for alleviating stress.

It's okay to soothe difficult emotions—it's not okay to do it with food (or alcohol or drugs). When you soothe difficult emotions with food, your mind-body system (your neurological system) creates neurological connections that, in turn, create strong urges to eat in response to emotional cues. This is *habit*. Habit says, "If a little is good, more is better." An addiction always asks for more of itself.

Sugar, starches, and alcohol enter the bloodstream rapidly because they are easily broken down in the digestive tract, so they bring fast "relief," and these are the substances that most people choose for emotional eating. These substances cross the blood-brain barrier rapidly, exciting the hypothalamus, which causes an onslaught of chemical messengers that go to cellular receptors. Cells have receptors for all sorts of chemicals. When receptors for starches, sugar, and alcohol are "turned on" repeatedly, the cells become conditioned to receive those kinds of chemicals—and to generate discomfort when those chemicals are withheld. This is addiction.[1] Recovering from any addiction is a long, arduous, often uncomfortable process, because it requires deprogramming the neurological system.

Reverse the Addiction to Food

Here are some ways to curb emotional eating and reverse your addiction to food.

---

1. For more education about neurochemistry, see the documentary *What the Bleep Do We Know?* by Captured Light Industries, available on DVD.

- Remove comfort foods from your home and replace them with healthful snacks.
- One way to reverse a habit is to replace it with another ritual. Turn to healthier ways to soothe difficult emotions.
- Negotiate with friends, coworkers, and family to support you and stop tempting you with sweets and fattening foods.
- When you are faced with the temptation of sugary, starchy foods, say NO immediately. Don't give yourself time to mull it over.
- Don't attend gatherings that focus on fattening foods—the wine and cheese party, the ice-cream social, the chocolate cake bake-off.
- Trying to taper off gradually doesn't work because it's easier to turn down the first cookie than the tenth—by then, you are "on a roll." Until you can effectively and consistently manage stress in healthy ways, it's best to avoid problem foods altogether, so that they are not even an option to consider.
- Be aware of the ways in which you sabotage yourself and STOP IT! Do you say, "Just this once is okay" or "Just one doughnut won't hurt" or "I am really down today, so this time doesn't count?"
- Believe you CAN reverse this addiction.
- Take it one day at a time. The reality you live with today won't be the reality of your entire life. Each morning when you wake up, tell yourself, "For today, I am willing to make the choices that promote my health and well-being."

You have to want something else more than you want food, even during times of discomfort. The question is not whether you want cheesecake right now, but whether you want to remain overweight. Every time you turn to food for comfort you make a statement that you are willing to remain overweight and continue feeling unhappy about it. Eating a slice of cheesecake should feel like an abhorrent transgression, an assault on your body, a violation of your values! Extreme weight gain is a serious threat to health, and emotional eating is a serious addiction. Serious health problems and addictions require extreme measures.

Expect to backslide from time to time. Don't get discouraged and, above all, don't give up! Just go back to whatever works and keep doing it. What are your problem foods? What are you going to do differently to stress-proof your life, improve your coping skills, and reverse your addiction to emotional eating?

Special Bonus Report for Session 4

Boost Your Brain to Curb Compulsive Eating!

According to neuropsychiatrist Daniel Amen, compulsive eating and binging may sometimes be symptoms of depression; fatigue; imbalance in blood sugars; chemical imbalances in the brain, such as reduced serotonin levels; or some combination of these factors. Amen writes that brain activity problems can be caused by a number of factors, including toxic substances, genetics, stress, trauma, high fevers, head injury, or a poor diet—even if some of these risk factors occurred much earlier in a person's life.[1] Dr. Amen has recently published several books on the interactions among brain chemistry, lifestyle, depression, compulsions, and anxiety, and many of his recommendations are described here. If you or a member of your family has a problem with compulsive eating, consider this brain-health advice:[2]

- Get a complete physical exam. Ideally, the exam should include tests for blood sugar, lipids and cholesterol levels (via blood sampling), and brain-activity patterns (via brain imaging).

- Take a daily multivitamin containing B complex vitamins at the dosage recommended on the label.

- Take 1,000 milligrams of fish oil or omega-3 fatty acids daily.

- Eliminate alcohol, nicotine, and illegal drugs. All these substances have the potential to damage the brain and may aggravate existing brain problems and emotional difficulties.

- Limit exposure to toxic chemicals, such as spray paints, insecticides, and so on.

- Studies show conclusively that inadequate sleep affects hormones associated with mood and appetite, and correlates with weight gain. Get eight hours of uninterrupted sleep each night. Avoid caffeine and stimulating activity late in the day. Drink milk (providing you are not lactose intolerant or allergic

---

1. D. G. Amen and L. C. Routh. *Healing Anxiety and Depression.* (New York: Berkeley Books, 2004).
2. These recommendations have been reviewed by a professional nutritionist. This report is not intended as a cure for any disease or as a substitute for medical advice. If symptoms are severe or persistent, consult a physician or mental-health professional.

to dairy products) or take melatonin (75 milligrams orally) at bedtime. Resting in a dark, quiet room may help with falling asleep. Do not take melatonin in combination with supplements containing magnesium or zinc.

- Switch to a diet high in protein, eating five or six small portions throughout the day.

- Choose complex carbohydrates (vegetables, fresh fruits, and whole grains) over-processed foods containing refined sugars and simple carbohydrates (white bread, baked goods, pasta, white rice, and potatoes). Consult a nutritionist as needed.

- Take Saint-John's-wort (for adults, 600 milligrams in the morning and 300 milligrams before bed). Saint-John's-wort is contraindicated for women who are taking birth-control pills or are pregnant or breast-feeding. When taking Saint-John's-wort, avoid foods and beverages containing tyramine, such as Chianti wine, beer, aged cheese, chicken livers, chocolate, bananas, and meat tenderizers. Avoid sun exposure. Caution: Saint-John's-wort may have adverse interactions with prescription antidepressants, lithium, alcohol, birth-control pills, cold and allergy drugs, flu medicines, decongestants, protease inhibitors for HIV, amphetamines, and narcotic pain relievers. Always consult a physician or pharmacist about the possible interactions between nutritional and herbal supplements and prescription or over-the-counter medications.

- L-tryptophan and 5-HTP are nutritional supplements that may boost serotonin levels in the brain. The recommended dosage for adults is 1,000 to 3,000 milligrams of L-tryptophan at bedtime and 50 to 100 milligrams of 5-HTP three times daily, with or without food. L-tryptophan may have an adverse interaction with antidepressants, lithium, and other prescription medications such as Imitrex and Ambien. Again, always consult a physician or pharmacist about the possible interactions between nutritional and herbal supplements and prescription or over-the-counter medications.

- Get adequate daily physical activity.

- Exposure to sunlight may also help (if you are not taking Saint-John's-wort). The brain seems to respond well to natural light. Sunlight activates vitamin D in the skin, which supports the brain's production of tryptophan—nature's own tranquilizer. Just use sunscreen to protect the skin from UV rays.

- If you have sleep problems or depression, consult a physician concerning the value and possible side-effects of prescription antidepressants and sleep-enhancing medications.

References

Amen, D. G., and L. C. Routh. 2004. *Healing Anxiety and Depression*. New York: Berkeley Books.

Gangwisch, J. et al. 2004. Lack of Sleep May Lead to Excess Weight. Paper presented to the North American Association for the Study of Obesity Annual Scientific Meeting, November 14–18, 2004, Las Vegas, Nevada. [Abstract 42-OR]

Mignot, E. et al. 2004. Stanford Study Links Obesity to Hormonal Changes from Lack of Sleep. *Public Library of Science*, Dec. 6. (Cited on Stanford University Medical Center, Office of Communication and Public Affairs web site.)

Taheri, S. 2004. The Mechanisms for the Interaction between Sleep and Metabolism. Available online at the University of Bristol, Laboratories for Integrative Neurosciences and Endocrinology web site <www.bris.ac.uk/neuroscience/research/research/groups/pidetails/105>.

Assignment for Session 5
A Two-Week Food Diary

Are you selecting and eating healthful foods on a daily basis, or are you going after fattening foods with little nutritional value? Everyone likes an indulgence food once in a while—as a special treat. Some people can handle that occasional treat and still maintain a healthy weight. They seem to have an internal monitoring system that automatically regulates their caloric intake. They might feel like eating a slice of chocolate cake one day, and then crave only celery the next day. At some level they are conscious of what they are eating and what it takes to sustain their weight at a consistent level that they like. They know what is fattening and tend to steer away from those foods and gravitate toward low-calorie, low-fat foods—and they don't feel deprived!

You can train yourself to think in this way, but it requires conscious effort in the beginning. The first step is to eat consciously and conscientiously, being more aware of what you put in your shopping cart, on your plate, and in your mouth. The following activity is designed to help you develop the habit of selecting healthful, nutritious food, as opposed to fattening foods that pile on the calories!

Activity: Healthful Foods and Not-So-Healthful Foods

Step 1

The first step will get you into the habit of making distinctions between fattening foods and slenderizing foods. The chart on the next page has two columns. In the column labeled "Not-So-Healthful Foods" make a list of foods and beverages you commonly eat that are high in sugars, salts, fats, and alcohol. In the column labeled "Healthful, Nutritious Foods" list foods and beverages (that you are willing to eat) that are low in sugars, salts, fats, and alcohol, but high in nutritional value, containing vitamins, minerals, protein, and fiber.

If you aren't sure how to categorize some foods, do your homework. Look at food labels and consult a nutrition guide or calorie counter. Don't be fooled by "combination foods." Steamed broccoli is a low-fat, nutritious food, unless you pour hollandaise sauce over it. A baked potato is a healthy food, until you smother it with butter, cheese, or sour cream. Fried foods have more fat and calories than those that are boiled, poached, steamed, grilled, or baked.

If there are more Not-So-Healthful Foods on your list than Healthful, Nutritious Foods, then perhaps you'll want (1) to expand your food selections to find more healthful foods that appeal to you, and (2) to find ways to cook and prepare healthful foods so that they taste better to you. There are plenty of low-fat cookbooks around that contain delicious recipes.

Step 2

For the next week, keep a food diary. Yes, it's a hassle, but so is being overweight! How else are you really going to be aware of how much and what you eat? Write down everything you eat—yes, everything—and the approximate numbers of calories you consume. Beside each item, note whether it is a Not-So-Healthful Food or a Healthful, Nutritious Food. The reason for this step is to help you become more aware of what you are eating, so that you really do have to stop and think about each type of food you select and make a conscious decision about it.

Even the act of keeping a record may change your food-selection habits, because you will be more aware of how you get yourself to choose Healthful or Not-So-Healthful foods. Try to catch yourself when you say, "Well, this one helping won't matter" or "Well, this one slice of cake won't hurt me" or "Just one more chocolate." Also notice when you make a good choice, and when you say to yourself, "Hmm, what will satisfy my appetite but is also good for me?"

Not-So-Healthful Foods	Healthful, Nutritious Foods

Step 3

At the end of week 1, review your food diary and answer these questions.

a. Did you really write down each thing you ate and the number of calories in it? If you did, good for you! Your motivation is strong! If you didn't, and you "cheated" a little, ask yourself why. Were you avoiding the truth? Did you say you didn't want to bother? Did you say it wouldn't matter anyway? Were you going easy on yourself? If so, then think about how these kinds of halfhearted attitudes might be showing up in other areas of your life. Those may be the same attitudes that led you to overeat and allowed you to put on all those extra pounds without doing anything about it sooner, when you weighed just four or five pounds too much.

b. Did your Not-So-Healthful Food calories outnumber your Healthful, Nutritious Food calories, or vice versa? If healthful food calories outnumbered not-so-healthful foods, congratulations! If not-so-healthful calories outnumbered healthful choices, then you may want to rethink your eating patterns. Strive for a four-to-one ratio of healthful calories to not-so-healthful calories. Choose unhealthful foods in small portions—sometimes a single bite will satisfy a craving.

c. How did you lead yourself to make not-so-healthful choices? What was the situation? What was your physical and emotional state? What did you tell yourself? What could you have done instead? What would it have taken from you to make better choices?

d. How did you get yourself to make healthful choices? Every time you made a healthful choice, what were two or three common success factors that led to the decision? Was one factor a feeling or a thought? An attitude? Something that happened earlier that day that affected your emotional state? Something you said to yourself, or maybe something you heard someone else say? Something about the food itself that you noticed? Did you go through a decision process in your mind? It's important that you identify those success factors—because they work! Those success factors, even if they occurred only a few times, are the source of your competence in making intelligence choices about food. Write them down on an index card so that you can remember them.

Step 4

Think ahead to the next week. Mentally walk through the upcoming days and imagine all those times and places where you could apply your success factors.

Imagine getting into the habit of using those success factors more and more often as you increase your healthful food choices.

Step 5

For week 2, keep a food diary again, and write down everything you eat and the approximate caloric value of each food or beverage. This week, however, make a conscious effort to apply your success factors whenever possible.

Step 6

At the end of week 2, review your food diary. Compare week 1 to week 2. Do you notice any differences? What was the difference that made the difference? What improvements or enhancements might you want to make to your success factors? What are you learning about making intelligent choices about food? What do you want to remember? What will you do now, in order to make consistently good food choices?

If week 2 wasn't an improvement over week 1, what happened? In what ways were you blocking your success? What got in the way? What were the setbacks? Were the setbacks things you could have handled differently? Did you notice anything you'd like to change in your thoughts, emotional responses, actions, or interactions with others? What are you more aware of now? What did you learn, and how will you apply that information, now and in the future? What will you do now, in order to enhance your ability to make consistently good food choices?

Why Are Food Choices Important?

Food choices are important because

1. Balanced nutrition requires a variety of foods that supply the body's needs for vitamins, minerals, amino acids, protein, fiber, water, starch, and fat.

2. Food is the body's source of energy. Energy is derived from calories. When caloric intake exceeds caloric metabolism (the rate at which the body burns calories), then the body stores those extra calories as body fat.

An ideal nutritional plan supplies nutrients mostly from low-calorie foods, to avoid excessive calories that result in extra body fat, which is a health risk. The following table shows the calories required to sustain a stable weight (without losing any weight).

Table 1. Daily caloric needs based on general activity level

General Activity Level	Women	Men
Sedentary: sitting most of day, with little physical activity.	Multiply body weight (in pounds) by 14 calories. For kilos, multiply by 31 calories.	Multiply body weight (in pounds) by 15 calories. For kilos, multiply by 33 calories.
Light activity: standing most of the day.	Multiply body weight (in pounds) by 15 calories. For kilos, multiply by 35 calories.	Multiply body weight (in pounds) by 16 calories. For kilos, multiply by 35 calories.
Moderate activity: daily activity includes walking, gardening, and housework.	Multiply body weight (in pounds) by 16 calories. For kilos, multiply by 40 calories.	Multiply body weight (in pounds) by 17 calories. For kilos, multiply by 47 calories.
High activity: dancing, skating, tennis, jogging, aerobics, or manual labor such as construction work or farmwork.	Multiply body weight (in pounds) by 17 calories. For kilos, multiply by 48 calories.	Multiply body weight (in pounds) by 19 calories. For kilos, multiply by 42 calories.
	Pregnant women: add 300 calories per day.	
	Lactating women: add 500 calories per day.	
	Women over 50: subtract 250 calories per day. (Reduced estrogen decreases metabolism.)	

Source: American Cancer Society: "Calculate Your Daily Needs." Available online at <www.cancer.org/docroot/PED/content/PED61xCalorieCalculator.asp?sitearea=&level=>. These numbers may vary slightly according to the source one consults. Individual calorie needs may also vary from those recommended here.

A-39

You don't always have to count calories, but calories do count. If you have a weight problem, it means you've been consuming more calories than your body is burning. The formula for weight reduction is simple (mathematically at least). You must burn more calories than you consume. That means, in order to lose weight, you must reduce caloric intake or increase calorie-burning activity or both. (Usually both because it can be difficult to meet your body's nutritional needs over the long term if you go for calorie reduction alone.) How many calories do you have to burn to achieve one pound in weight reduction? A whopping 3,500 calories!

To reduce one pound in seven days, you could, in theory, lower your caloric intake by 500 calories a day, or put forth extra physical effort sufficient to burn 500 calories a day. The amount of calories burned depends on the type of activity. The amount of sustained activity required to burn approximately 500 calories would be

- 30 minutes of walking up stairs or skiing on a skiing machine
- 60 minutes of jogging, aerobic dancing, skipping rope, tennis, or bicycling
- 120 minutes of swimming, horseback riding, dancing, badminton, or volleyball
- 150 minutes of walking, housework, or yard work

Exercise is a must because it builds muscle, burns calories, and increases metabolism. Although burning off 500 calories a day is doable, such a regimen is too extreme for most individuals. If the 500-calorie reduction comes only from less food, the lower calorie intake may trigger the body's energy-conservation response. The body gets the idea that it may starve and slows metabolism, so calorie burning is less efficient. A reduction of 250 calories a day is less likely to trigger the energy-conservation response. At a calorie-reduction and burn rate of 250 calories a day, you could drop one pound in two weeks. Remember, as your weight goes down, your body requires fewer calories per day, so you continue to subtract 250 calories from progressively lower daily calorie requirements. Given that you want balanced nutrition while lowering caloric intake, the best approach is to get daily physical activity and choose healthful foods in moderate quantities.

Assignment for Session 6
The NLP Slender Eating Strategy

This strategy will help you develop a healthy relationship with food, eat sensibly, and curb a tendency to eat because of emotions or external triggers. This adaptation of the NLP Naturally Slender Eating Strategy is a way to make decisions about food, eating, and hunger in the same way a Trim-Slim person would—except that a Trim-Slim person does so automatically, without conscious thought. The procedure was originally developed by NLP trainers Connirae and Steve Andreas and is described in their book *Heart of the Mind*.

Instructions: Apply this variation of the NLP Naturally Slender Eating Strategy at least once a day for the next week. You can use it during a snack or an entire meal.

Step 1

When you feel the urge to eat something, stop whatever you are doing at the moment. Sit down and get quiet with yourself. Concentrate on your inner responses. Ask yourself what is prompting you to eat at this moment.

- Is it some cue in your environment, such as the sight or smell of food, the time of day, or talk about food?
- Is it some emotion, such as boredom, disappointment, anger, anxiety, worry, fear, guilt, loneliness, or disappointment?
- Is it because you don't like yourself right now, or don't like your life right now?
- Is it that you feel happy and you are celebrating something, or perhaps you want to reward yourself?
- Or is it that you truly feel hungry: your stomach is empty, and your body needs an energy boost?

If your answer falls in one of the first four categories, be aware that your desire to eat is due not to hunger, but to something else. You now have a choice. Decide if you really want food, or if there is something else you want. You are learning to distinguish hunger from other eating triggers. If you decide you aren't really hungry, and you choose to do something other than eat, you can stop the process here. Otherwise, if you really are hungry, or you really do need an energy boost, go on to step 2.

Step 2

If you've decided to eat something, this step will help you decide what to eat. Concentrate on the sensations in your mouth and stomach. In the beginning you might find it helpful to close your eyes for this step and to place the palm of your hand on your stomach area, just below your rib cage. Ask yourself, "What would taste good in my mouth and feel good in my stomach right now?" Think over the foods that are available to you and acceptable to you. You might be thinking about what you have on hand in the kitchen if you are at home, or about what is on the menu if you are in a restaurant.

Step 3

Think of a food (or combination of foods) you could eat. Now imagine eating a serving of that food. Think about how the food will taste and feel in your mouth, how it will feel as you swallow it. Does it seem that this food (or food combination) will be satisfying, in terms of smell, taste, and texture? If not, think of another possibility. Test out the options in your mind until you find an acceptable food that will satisfy your mouth.

Step 4

Now think about how much of this food (or combination of foods) you want to eat. Again, place your hand on your stomach, close your eyes, and ask yourself, "How much of this food will give me a satisfied feeling of fullness in my stomach? Do I want just a small portion to fill a small space, a medium-sized portion to fill a medium space, or a full meal to fill my whole stomach?" Sometimes you can get an intuitive indication, before eating, of just how much you want to eat. Remember, the average adult human stomach can comfortably hold only about two heaping handfuls of food—that should give you a starting point. If this step doesn't work for you, don't worry. Just take a small portion for now and go on to the next step.

Step 5

Think about how you will feel immediately after you have eaten this food in this amount. Think about how you will feel an hour afterward. Will you feel satisfied? Will you feel guilty? Will you wish you had eaten something else? If you anticipate feeling guilt or regret, maybe your food choice isn't the best you could make. Go back to step 2 and start again. Consider other choices. When you have a choice that will leave you satisfied, without guilt or regret, then go on to step 6.

Step 6

Now begin to eat slowly and attentively, concentrating your attention on each bite. It's ideal to do this exercise alone. If you are with a companion and want to have a conversation, however, just put your fork down between bites, while you talk. Taking a drink of water between bites is another way to eat more slowly.

While you are eating, pause every few bites, put down your fork, and breathe deeply. At each pause, focus your attention on the feeling in your stomach. Again, you might want to place the palm of your hand on your stomach, pressing in gently. Notice the difference in the way your stomach feels now, with food in it, compared to how it did when you first began this exercise, with no or little food in your stomach. Remain aware of the feeling in your stomach as you continue to eat slowly. It might even help to picture the amount of food you have eaten, as it begins to take up the space in your stomach. Continue eating until you are aware of that comfortable, not-quite-full feeling. Now pause for a minute to notice whether that not-quite-full feeling develops into a comfortably full feeling in your stomach. If not, take another bite and wait a minute. Keep taking one bite at a time until you get that satisfied, full feeling. You might notice other changes, too—perhaps a sense of contentment or more mental alertness, depending on what you've eaten.

Step 7

When you are aware of that full feeling, stop eating. Put your fork down and push your plate away. It doesn't matter if there is food left on it or if someone offers you a second helping. It doesn't matter if someone else encourages you to eat more. Just say, "No thanks. I've eaten enough and I don't want any more. I'm not hungry now." Get up and leave the table or, if you are in a restaurant, ask the wait staff to remove your plate.

Feel a sense of accomplishment that you are learning to eat according to your body's communications. Soon you will develop the habit of eating healthful foods when you feel hungry, in just the right amount to satisfy your hunger, and you'll stop eating when you feel full.

When You've Completed This Exercise

When you've practiced this exercise once a day for a week, think about everything you learned and answer the following questions.

• What steps of the process worked for you?

- For the steps of the process that worked for you, how did they help?
- Is there some way you could modify this process to better meet your needs?
- What improvements in your eating habits did you notice over the course of the week?

Now envision that over the next few days and weeks you are applying what you learned from this assignment as you enhance your relationship with food, and you find that you are making progress toward your preferred weight.

The Naturally Slender Eating Strategy was developed by NLP trainers and practitioners Connirae and Steve Andreas and is described in Heart of the Mind, *by Connirae Andreas and Steve Andreas (Moab, UT: Real People Press, 1989).*

Assignment for Session 7
Mind Management

Making lifestyle changes requires changes in how you think. The way you think is important because your thoughts determine how you feel and how you act. Your emotions and actions determine whether you remain overweight and unhappy with your size and shape, or whether you reduce that weight and have the size and shape you prefer.

I hope by now you are thinking positive, productive, motivating thoughts—especially those thoughts that prompt you to exercise regularly and to maintain an intelligent relationship with food. If you are still having problems with negative, pessimistic thinking, low self-esteem, self-criticism, or discouragement, however, then this assignment will prove especially helpful to you.

Manage your mind and you manage your life! How you think is your responsibility! You are not stuck with bad internal programming. Learn to run your mind efficiently and effectively, and you'll never be fat again! Running your mind in this way requires that you put a stop to negative, defeating self-talk; change your internal imagery; focus your attention in new ways; examine and evaluate how you are living your life; and instill a positive, motivating, uplifting dialogue. In effect, you learn to "quality control" what goes on in your mind, so that your thoughts support your outcomes consistently. Let's examine these ways to manage your mind.

Put a Stop to Negative, Defeating Self-Talk

Here are four methods you can use to put a stop to negative internal dialogue that criticizes you, sabotages you, depresses you, and steers you wrong every time.[1] The four methods are reframing, refuting, refusal, and replacement. Use these methods consistently and soon your negative self-talk will be extinguished.

Reframing: Reframing is a way to change meaning. Listen carefully to the negative things you are saying to yourself to determine whether there is an underlying positive intention. In other words, maybe the message is negative, but the

---

1. These methods are summarized in *Brain Lock: Free Yourself from Obsessive-Compulsive Behavior*, by Jeffrey Schwartz, M.D., and Beverly Beyette, M.D. (New York: HarperCollins, 1997).

underlying intent is positive. If so, find something else to say to yourself to satisfy the intention without the negative language. Suppose you've been saying to yourself, "I'm too clumsy to exercise." Then you realize the positive intention is a desire to be safe, based on a fear that you might accidentally injure yourself with strenuous exercise. Change your internal dialogue to, "I exercise safely and sensibly."

Refuting: When you say something negative and irrational to yourself, convince yourself that the negative message just isn't true—and, in fact, it's silly and ridiculous. Give yourself the evidence to refute the negative, irrational statement.

Refusal: Refuse to entertain the negative messages. Refuse to dwell on them. Tell them, "No, I don't care what you say. I'm not listening, and I give no credence to any of this nonsense." Imagine that your mind is like a radio that can play a lot of different kinds of music, based on where you set the dial. If you don't like what's going on in your mind, turn the dial to a new frequency.

Replacement: Replace and counter each negative message with a positive message, immediately.

Problem behaviors develop because of problematic thinking. Isn't it strange that so many people are reluctant to think positive thoughts such as "I love and respect my body," yet are eager to think negative thoughts such as "I'll always be fat, and there is nothing I can do about it"? Those kinds of thoughts keep people stuck and perpetuate unhealthful patterns. Every thought, negative or positive, is a direct instruction to the mind-body neurology, which strives to make those thoughts come true.

Change Your Internal Imagery

What movies do you play in your mind? What pictures are you looking at? Do you replay depressing movies of defeat and disappointment? Do you see yourself as a fat person for life? Do you obsess about food and drool over Technicolor mental images of fattening foods? Images are a form of thought. Change your imagery to healthful images with positive meanings. Can you imagine how you'll look once you have your preferred weight? Can you see yourself fitting into the same size you wore in high school, dancing at the high school reunion? Can you picture the look of astonishment on the face of an old friend (or better yet, an ex-boyfriend or girlfriend) who says, "Wow, what happened? You look great!" Every accomplishment begins with an idea in the mind.

WHY Client Workbook © 2006 Crown House Publishing, www.CHPUS.com, www.crownhouse.co.uk

Focus Your Attention in New Ways

Where do you direct your attention? Put down the dessert cookbook, with the full-page color photos of luscious-looking desserts, and pick up a book on health and fitness. Pass up the candy aisle and the bakery section in the supermarket. Nothing there interests you now. Steer yourself over to the produce department and really look at the gorgeous colors of those fruits and vegetables. Enjoy the smells. Leave your TV and computer alone for a while and go for a walk in the sunshine. Stop feeling down and go do something you enjoy. Why dwell on hurts and anger? Are you focusing on the problem or on the solution? Do you focus on your weaknesses or on your strengths? Whatever you focus your attention on becomes something you do more often or choose more often. Stop focusing on the things that made you overweight and pay attention to the things that keep you healthy.

Examine How You Are Living Your Life

Are you hard on yourself? Do you criticize yourself because you are not perfect? Do you let mistakes and setbacks stall your progress? Do you berate yourself because you don't have the body of a starlet, or even the body you had when you were eighteen? Do you compare yourself to other people and then feel disappointed? Even when you have a success, do you discount it and say, "Oh well, that was just one time—it doesn't count." Do you feel bad about yourself because you wait for praise and recognition from others—and either it isn't forthcoming, or when you get it, you brush it off or think it isn't enough? Maybe it's time to straighten out your thinking in terms of expectations, beliefs, and values.

Overeating and binging are no substitutes for a fulfilling life and for following your passions. Being overweight is similar to living with a disability. In your case, you can change it, but doing so is hard work.

Start out by looking at the big picture of your life. Are you just muddling through life haphazardly, waiting for something good to happen, or are you following plans that fulfill your dreams? What are you living for? Do you have a purpose that gives your life meaning? What activities bring you fulfillment, challenge you, and call forth your talents? What are you doing to break through external restrictions and internal inhibitions so that you are living your life in a way that is enriching and rewarding? Are you planning? Are you setting your outcomes? Are you getting beneficial help and support? When you have ready, affirmative answers to these questions, you will be too busy, too excited, too engaged in the triumphs and struggles of living to even think about food!

Life has far more to offer than chocolate bars and French fries—but you have to want it, work for it, sweat the details, and persist, despite the setbacks, obstacles, and opposition. You have to decide what's really important and worthwhile and stop settling for less. Believe that your happiness, health, and contentment are worth the effort it takes to achieve what's important to you. Then align your actions with your plans, values, and beliefs—then food becomes a mere distraction—and having to put up with the inconvenience of excess weight is a waste of time and energy.

Now look at the various aspects of your life. Examples are

- identity, personal growth and self-development
- family life
- social life and friendships
- mental and physical health
- career and education
- finances
- spirituality
- leisure, hobbies, home life, and recreation
- community involvement and civic participation.

Obviously, some of these areas are more important to you than others. Nevertheless, these aspects of living are where you put your time, money, and energy. For each one, rate your satisfaction with yourself on a scale from 1 to 10. Although few people will rate their lives a 10 in every area, the areas with low ratings will indicate where the pain and disappointments in your life exist. What would it take to raise a low rating by 1 point, say from a 4 to a 5? What aspects of your life could use improvement, and what actions could you take to implement those improvements? Devise a plan. Lifestyle improvements are not easy, and they don't happen overnight. With consistent effort and discipline, you will see results.

Install a Positive, Uplifting Dialogue

How do you talk to yourself to uplift your spirit, give yourself motivation and encouragement, stay productive, cope with challenges, and boost your self-esteem? Do you talk to yourself in the manner of a loving friend and an expert coach? You should! After you've cleared out all that nasty, negative self-criticism, what do you say instead? Develop the vocabulary of personal encouragement and self-love. Stand in front of a mirror, look yourself squarely in the eye, and say, "I love you!" Learn to comfort yourself with words instead of food. Be your own cheering squad. Whenever you do something right, cheer yourself on. Enumerate your finer qualities and accomplishments to yourself on a regular basis. Give yourself permission to be healthy, happy, fulfilled, confident, successful, and beautiful. Sing your favorite songs. Spend five minutes a day feeling grateful. Call yourself "sweetheart" and pamper yourself. Stop being a martyr and a doormat. When you face a new challenge say, "I can do this. I can figure this out."

During hypnosis, in session 8 of the WHY program, you can add words of encouragement that you want your practitioner to say to you—things that you want to remember so that you will continue to practice healthful eating patterns and remain physically active. List the sentences that you want to hear in the space below.

Words of Encouragement

_____

_____

_____

_____

_____

_____

_____

Another way to install a positive, uplifting dialogue in your head is to develop affirmations and repeat them to yourself frequently. Affirmations are a way to program your mind for success. An affirmation is a short declarative statement that shapes beliefs and attitudes. "I choose healthful low-fat foods and enjoy them," is an example.

No one is completely sure how affirmations work. Some psychologists hypothesize that repeated ideas and actions (negative or positive) form neurological connections in the brain that, after a time, become "hard wired" to the point that they function automatically. This is how habits form. Some adhere to the theory of psycho-cybernetics, which states that frequently repeated thoughts eventually become imprinted on the subconscious mind, thus becoming a self-fulfilling prophecy.

Affirmations should be personal, reflecting your goals and values. They should be about you, with words such as "I" and "me" and "my." Your affirmations could start with the words "I am ...," "I have ... ," or "I do ... ." It's a good idea

A-49

to state affirmations in the present tense, the reason being that if your affirmations are stated in future tense ("I will …"), then the subconscious mind feels no urgency to act upon them now. If you think it's disingenuous to state your affirmations in the present tense (as in "I am slender and healthy"), then state your affirmations as a process (as in "I am becoming more slender and healthier each day").

Make your affirmations believable and realistic, so that you can say them with sincerity. Begin with small, achievable goals and work up to bigger accomplishments. "I am a world-class athlete" is a fine affirmation, but "I walk a mile each day" is probably more believable. Make your affirmations short, catchy, and easy to remember. "I like myself" is better than "I am now achieving the psychological state of self-esteem and personal dignity that fosters my well-being and is essential to mental health."

Make affirmations a part of your daily routine. Write them on index cards and post them in prominent places—on your bathroom mirror or the dashboard of your car. Set them to music and sing them. Say them aloud while driving or walking. Write them in a journal. Have your favorite one printed on a T-shirt.

When you learned self-hypnosis in session 3, you were encouraged to use affirmations in your self-hypnosis templates. During session 8, you will have the opportunity to specify affirmations that you want included in your hypnotherapy session. Use the space below to list the affirmations you want to hear. Remember to take this list with you when you meet with your practitioner for session 8.

Your Affirmations

_____

_____

_____

_____

_____

_____

Search Your Heart and Soul

Every problem has something to teach us about ourselves. To some extent, our bodies are metaphors for the way we live our lives. Are you holding on to resentment, anger, pain, or fear from the past? Are you, for example, stuffing emotions inside or swallowing anger you are afraid to express? Are you using excess weight to shield yourself from some threat that no longer exists—or maybe one you need to confront? Does your preoccupation with food and weight problems prevent you from addressing an issue you need to resolve once and for all? Does being overweight allow you to avoid a responsibility? Does your weight say something for you that you are afraid to say for yourself? Is there some issue with which you need to come to terms? Journaling on these questions may help you come up with the answers.

Perhaps some introspection and emotional healing will free you from the diet-and-binge cycle once and for all. If you think your weight problems are tied to some heavy emotional issues, you don't have to go it alone. Find a good counselor or psychotherapist to work with. Perhaps your WHY Program practitioner can schedule additional sessions to work with you on these emotional issues, or could refer you to a colleague.

Tend the Garden of Your Mind

Think of your mind as a garden and of yourself as the gardener. You are in charge of what grows in your garden. Do you want lovely, fragrant flowers, or do you want weeds? The quality of your "mind garden" determines the kind of results you'll get in accomplishing your goals. Weed out the negative thoughts and nurture thoughts that inspire productivity, motivation, discipline, and accomplishment. Value your thoughts and keep them positive, caring, and productive.

Decades ago, the philosopher Descartes wrote, "Cogito, ergo sum" ("I think, therefore I am"). If, indeed, the act of thinking is a measure of existence, then surely an interplay exists between the quality of our thoughts and the quality of our lives. When you are managing your mind, you are no longer at war with yourself. You are living your values and wishes congruently and authentically, with personal integrity.

Portions of this assignment were excerpted and adapted from "How You Can Benefit from Self-Talk" by Judith E. Pearson, which appeared in The Toastmaster, *January 1993.*

Special Bonus Report for Session 7
The Benefits of Exercise

If all the benefits of exercise could be squeezed into a pill, it would be considered a miracle drug—the "rejuvenation pill." Everyone would want it and would be willing to pay thousands of dollars for the extraordinary advantages—which come with no side-effects! No one would want to be without it. So why don't more people get off their behinds and exercise?

Newspapers, books, television shows, and magazines extol the benefits of physical exercise and activity as a means to physical fitness and a longer life. In every town and city in the United States you can find bike paths, jogging trails, health clubs, gyms, racquet clubs, tennis courts, aerobics classes, dance studios, martial arts classes, and community recreation facilities. You would surmise that the country is caught up in a frenzy of fitness. Although it is true that our population values exercise more than ever before, it is also true that obesity has reached epidemic proportions in this land of abundance and affluence. One-third of the population is overweight. In Black and Hispanic cultures and in low-income groups, 50 percent of the women are obese. Life doesn't have to be that way—and you don't have to be in the "fat people" category.

Regular exercise brings more than an improved physique. Exercise can help you *sleep better, manage stress more effectively, strengthen your heart, prevent osteoporosis, burn calories, decrease your appetite, improve your skin, and bolster your self-esteem*—and even more! WOW! Physical activity, combined with good nutrition, can actually slow the aging process itself. Let's look more closely at the rewards of exercise.

Exercise conditions your body to function more efficiently. The physical benefits of exercise are

Improved circulation, a stronger heart, and improved lung capacity: Aerobic activity works the heart muscle, increases blood flow, and makes the lungs pump harder—strengthening the entire cardiovascular system.

Healthier skin: Exercise increases circulation, bringing blood flow to the skin surface, carrying nutrients and flushing away toxins. Your skin looks younger, has a glow, and is healthier.

Prevention of osteoporosis: Weight-bearing exercises, such as walking, strengthen bones and can slow down bone loss due to aging.

Increased metabolism: Exercise burns calories and keeps the metabolic rate high for hours, even after the activity has ended.

Increased muscle tone: If you are dieting and reducing your food intake without exercising, you are losing muscle instead of fat. Muscle burns many more calories than fat, by a ratio of thirty to one. In order to retain muscle, you must exercise. Muscle weighs more than fat, but the tissue is denser and takes up less space, so you look slimmer as you build muscle tissues and burn more calories stored in fat.

Rehabilitation from muscular-skeletal injuries: Under the supervision of a sports physician or physical therapist, targeted exercises and movement can facilitate repair of damaged muscles, ligaments, and tendons. Sometimes even old injuries can improve with the proper exercise.

Exercise also gives you these psychological benefits:

Relief from stress and mild, transitory depression: Studies show that people who exercise have less stress. Exercise is a healthy way to work off frustration and anger. It gives "time out" from the demands of work and family. Increased circulation pumps oxygen to the brain for clearer thinking. Activities involving the whole body activate neurological activity across both hemispheres of the brain, which can have a calming effect.

Regulation of brain chemistry: A study by Nora Volkow, reported in the November–December 2004 issue of *Psychology Today*,[1] found that the brains of obese people are deficient in dopamine—a chemical involved in motivation, pleasure, and learning. The deficiency creates a "craving for stimulation" that prompts overeating and other addictions. As the addictive response develops over time, the prefrontal cortex, the part of the brain associated with judgment and inhibition, stops functioning normally. The antidote is prolonged, regular exercise, which causes the brain to release endorphins and elevates dopamine levels. Endorphins are the brain's own "feel good" chemicals (the release of endorphins causes the "runner's high" experienced by distance runners).

Increased self-esteem: Meeting a physical challenge—like finishing a ten-kilometer race or hiking a mountain trail or swimming twenty laps in a pool—brings the exhilaration of accomplishment and an enhanced sense of competence and mastery. Some people enjoy the camaraderie and fellowship of team sports and the shared fun of group activity. Some enjoy the improved grace that comes from activities involving precision movement such as dance, swimming, or gymnastics. Exercise can enhance your sense of self-worth.

---

1. K. McGowan. Addiction: Pay attention. *Psychology Today*, Nov.–Dec. 2004. Available online: Document ID 3571 <www.psychologytoday.com/articles/pto-3571.html>.

There is no pill, no medical treatment, no cosmetic preparation that can equal the benefits of regular physical exercise. Given these fantastic benefits, you can't pass it up! Exercise is absolutely essential to your health and well-being!

How to Get Started on an Exercise Routine

If you are not yet into an exercise routine, here are some ways to get started on a sensible regimen that will transform your mind, body, and spirit! The key to success is to set reasonable, incremental goals for yourself, so that you build strength and stamina slowly and safely over time. Follow these guidelines to developing an exercise routine:

Consult with your physician first: Get a complete physical exam and ask your physician about the types of exercise that are safe for you.

Choose a mix of activities: Ideally, you want an exercise routine that includes stretching exercises for flexibility, aerobic activity for cardiovascular fitness, and resistance exercises for strength and toning.

Consider a trainer: For optimal results, consult with a personal trainer who can help you design an exercise routine based on your age, physical condition, and fitness goals. A trainer is especially important if you plan to use weights or exercise machines. A personal trainer can help you start out at the proper speed and level of resistance, show you the proper postures and movements, and teach you how to avoid injury.

Get the right gear: Make sure you are wearing the proper clothing for your activity—that might mean footwear, protective knee pads, gloves, helmet, or a jogging bra or athletic supporter. If you use equipment, it should be in excellent condition and well maintained.

Warm up and stretch: At the beginning of your routine, spend about five minutes warming up—for example, walking in place or freestyle dancing—to get the blood circulating to your muscles and to loosen up your joints. Then stretch slowly until you feel some resistance and hold each stretch for a count of ten to twenty seconds. Warming up helps avoid muscle sprains.

Start slowly and pay attention to your body's responses: During the first days and weeks of a new exercise routine, be careful and don't push too hard. Limit your initial workouts to a few minutes of light activity—or to a few minutes more than you usually do. If you feel fatigue or pain, stop and rest and try again tomorrow. Build strength and stamina over several weeks or months, and increase the demands on your body gradually.

Make it fun: Do exercise you enjoy. Exercise alone in the privacy of your home or with a friend or go to a gym or join a class. If you think your routine is getting dull, build in some variety. Exercise to music, walk with your pooch, bicycle with your child, watch TV while you work out, take dance lessons with your spouse—the list is endless.

Chart your progress: Put a chart on your refrigerator that shows how many sit-ups you do each day or how many miles you walk or how many minutes you spend on the treadmill. Or just put a big gold star on the calendar for every day you exercise. Soon you will like what you see!

Integrate movement into your daily routine: You'll get more from exercise (and burn additional calories) if you move around and stay active during the day. If you sit most of the day, take breaks at least every hour and stand up, stretch, take a few deep breaths, and walk around for a few minutes.

Make an appointment with yourself for exercise time, and give that time top priority. Keep the appointment, as if it were an appointment to receive a million dollars or meet with world leaders or interview for your dream job or go on a date with someone you adore. Get into a daily routine, so you actually begin to look forward to exercising. Don't miss it for anything except an emergency. Don't let others talk you out of it. Make exercise time sacred and non-negotiable. Exercise is for you, to make you feel good and look good, and you are worth it!

Portions of this report were excerpted and adapted from Healthy Habits: Total Conditioning for a Healthy Body and Mind, *by Kathy Corsetty and Judith E Pearson (Lincoln, NE: Dageforde Press, 2000).*

Assignment for Session 8

Keep Going: Make Changes Last, Make Motivation Last

By this time, you've completed the eight sessions of the WHY Weight Reduction Program. You are improving your skills in many areas:

- defining your outcomes
- confronting your methods of self-sabotage and turning them around in positive directions
- learning self-hypnosis methods for working with your subconscious mind
- developing strategies for stress management and alternatives to emotional eating
- choosing healthful, nutritious foods instead of fattening foods
- eating less food than before but still feeling satisfied
- becoming more mindful of calorie counts
- getting into the habit of eating for nutrition, eating when you feel truly hungry, and stopping when you feel full
- adhering to the NLP Slender Eating Strategy and Slim-Trim Thinking
- developing a safe exercise regimen that you can enjoy.

You have begun to adopt a healthier lifestyle, and you are reducing your weight in healthful ways. Naturally, you want to maintain your momentum and motivation so that you reach and maintain your target weight. You want to make these changes last, so that you can look back at old photos of yourself when you were fat and say, *"Never again!"* Here are some recommendations to help you maintain your progress and stay on track with your weight-reduction efforts.

- Write a list of everything that is lovely, beautiful, and healthy about your body. Write a letter thanking your body for everything it has done for you. Write a promise to your body that you are going to achieve and maintain a healthy weight.

- Each day, take some quiet time to visualize yourself at your preferred weight, feeling and looking confident and self-assured, moving about easily, fitting into attractive, smaller-sized clothing. See yourself doing things you didn't do before when you were overweight—maybe exercising, dancing, bending over to tie your shoes, fitting comfortably into an airline seat.

A-57

- Each day, say positive affirmations to yourself that support your new lifestyle and your capacity to live your life as a Slim-Trim Person.

- Continue to plan your meals and set aside time for exercise sessions in advance so that they become routine and you are less likely to be side-tracked or distracted by temptations.

- The moment you see any extra pounds, take stock and take action. Are old habits creeping back in? Figure out where you got off-track and take action to reduce those excess pounds. Don't fall into denial and tell yourself it's okay and those extra pounds will go away by themselves. It's *not* okay, and putting on extra pounds is a slippery slope that will eventually demolish all your efforts. Do something about them *now*! Look again at your food intake and level of physical activity. You might even want to consult your physician to check for thyroid activity, hormone levels, insulin levels, and other chemical imbalances that may be contributing to weight gain.

- When you want to indulge, pamper, or soothe yourself, choose alternatives to food and dining out. Take a hot bath, get a massage, take a walk, read a good book, sleep in, chat with a friend, buy yourself a gift, take a day off—just don't overeat.

- Learn to say no and mean it. When someone offers you dessert or second helpings, say, "No, thank you." When someone asks you to babysit on your night at the gym, say, "I'd love to some other time, but not tonight."

- Negotiate with friends and loved ones for their support in maintaining your healthful lifestyle. If you need an evening away from the kids to go the gym, negotiate with your spouse to stay home with them. Maybe your roommate "surprises" you by cooking fattening meals or goodies and expecting you to eat them. Negotiate for a more sensible menu.

- Don't be afraid to waste food. It's better to waste food outside your body than inside your body. Leave it on your plate, save it for another meal, or throw it out instead of eating extra calories you don't need.

- When you eat in restaurants, look for items on the menu marked as low-fat or "heart healthy" meals. Unfortunately, many restaurants now serve over-sized helpings that are so big not even a hippopotamus could eat it all. If you are eating with others, ask someone to split a meal (or at least a main course) with you. Another strategy is to ask the waiter to bring a takeout box to the table and put half the meal into it, before you start to eat. Then eat what you have on your plate and have the takeout later.

- Listen to the WHY Weight Reduction Program recordings often. Read over the take-home assignments from time to time. Return to your practitioner for "booster" sessions if you need them.

Stay the course. Don't give up. Good luck. Celebrate a new, healthier version of you!

Index

Lightning Source UK Ltd.
Milton Keynes UK
UKHW03f0833110618
324036UK00005B/130/P